AF333548

FLUOROURACIL

SYNTHESIS, HEALTH EFFECTS AND ROLE IN CHEMOTHERAPY

PHARMACOLOGY - RESEARCH, SAFETY TESTING AND REGULATION

Additional books in this series can be found on Nova's website
under the Series tab.

Additional e-books in this series can be found on Nova's website
under the e-books tab.

CANCER ETIOLOGY, DIAGNOSIS AND TREATMENTS

Additional books in this series can be found on Nova's website
under the Series tab.

Additional e-books in this series can be found on Nova's website
under the e-books tab.

PHARMACOLOGY - RESEARCH, SAFETY TESTING AND REGULATION

FLUOROURACIL

SYNTHESIS, HEALTH EFFECTS AND ROLE IN CHEMOTHERAPY

ALBERTO C. DÁRIO LONGINHO
AND
SEBASTIAO E. BRITTO DOBREIRO
EDITORS

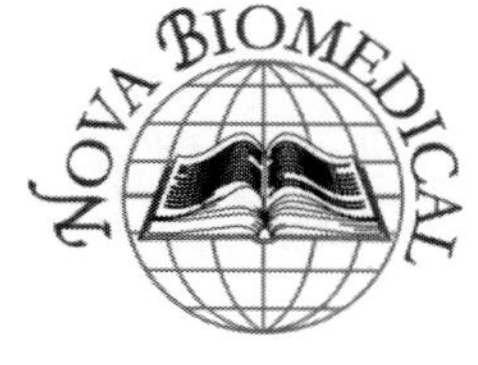

Nova Science Publishers, Inc.
New York

Library of Congress Cataloging-in-Publication Data

Library of Congress Control Number: 2012938174
ISBN: 978-1-62081-970-8

Published by Nova Science Publishers, Inc. † New York

CONTENTS

PREFACE

The fluoropyrimidine 5-fluorouracil (5-FU), an antimetabolite drug, works by being incorporated in the RNA and DNA and by the inhibition of the nucleotide synthetic enzyme thymidylate synthase. It is widely used in the treatment of a range of cancers, including gastrointestinal, head and neck, and breast cancers. In this book, the authors present current research in the study of the synthesis, health effects and role in chemotherapy of fluorouracil. Topics discussed include the antiproliferative activities, cell-cycle regulation, apoptosis and cellular differentiation of acyclic 5-fluorouracil O, N-Acetals; 5-fluorouracil and its immunotoxicity and side effects; 5-fluorouracil application in the management of bleb failure; and cisplatin and 5-fluorouracil for the treatment of ovarian adenocarcinoma.

Chapter II - The goal of cancer chemotherapy with classical drugs is often complicated by significant toxicity. As an alternative, induced differentiation modulates the cell programme by transforming malignant cells into mature cells with no proliferative potential. Our data demonstrate that (*RS*)-1-{[3-(2-hydroxyethoxy)-1-*iso*propoxy]propyl}-5-fluorouracil inhibits proliferation, induces myogenic differentiation and increases the expression of proteins specifically present in normally differentiated skeletal muscle cells against the rhabdomyosarcoma cell line RD. From a designing point of view, a benzene ring was fused to the side chain in order to increase the lipophilicity of the molecules. Herein we report the preparation and biological activity of three compounds being (*RS*)-1-[2-(5-substituted-2-hydroxybenzyloxy)-1-methoxyethyl]-5-fluorouracils. A catechol-derived compound and two salicyl-derived compounds such as (*RS*)-(*Z*)-1-[4-(2-hydroxyphenyl)-1-methoxy-but-3-enyl]-5-fluorouracil [(*Z*)-43] and its dihydrogenated derivative (*RS*)-1-[4-(2-hydroxyphenyl)-1-methoxybutyl]-5-fluorouracil were prepared to complete the set of six *O,N*-acetals. The most active compound against the MCF-7 breast cancer cell line was (*Z*)-43 (IC$_{50}$ = 9.40 ± 0.64 μM). Differentiated breast cancer cells generate fat deposits within the cytoplasm. The MCF-7 cells treated with (*Z*)-43 caused an increase in the lipid content over control cells after 3 days of treatment. Our results suggest that there may be significant potential advantages in the use of this new differentiating agent for the treatment of breast cancer.

Chapter II - 5-FU (5-fluorouracil, sold as Adrucil), a pyrimidine analog, has been widely used in the treatment of various cancers, including breast cancer, colorectal cancer, and cancers of digestive tract. Despite serious toxicity and considerable side effects, such as cardiotoxicity, ocular toxicity, hepatotoxicity and haematological toxicity, it is one of the first cancer treatments due to lack of better treatment options. Analogs of 5-FU have been studied as antimycotic, antimalarial, antineoplastic, antibacterial and antiviral (anti-HIV and anti- HBV) and anticancer agents. Newer analogs of 5-FU may prove effective and safe alternate of 5-FU for cancer treatment, in addition to their use in other diseases/disorders.

Chapter III - 5-Fluorouracil (5-FU), a fluorinated pyrimidine that belongs to the group of antimetabolites, has become a component of the standard therapy for a variety of solid tumors, including gastrointestinal, head and neck, and breast cancers. The common clinical toxicity of 5-FU is affect the *rapidly dividing tissues* such as the bone marrow hematopoietic cells, which induces an important immunosuppression that potentially causes infection easily and reduced anticancer immunity. In this chapter, the clinical immunological effects of 5-FU, as well as experimental models used to assess and identify new compounds to treat 5-FU-induced immunotoxicity, were summarized. Experimentally, peripheral hematological and bone marrow analysis, cytokines quantification, and histological examination of the thymus, spleen, and lymphoid organs have been used to assess the immunosuppression in 5-FU-treated animals. Different compounds have been described in literature as agents able to prevent/reduce 5-FU-induced immunotoxicity, including chitosans and polysaccharides. In summary, these data should be used to establish new directions and new goals in future research.

Chapter IV - Fluorouracil is a fluorinated pyrimidine anti-metabolite that functions as an anti-neoplastic agent by blocking DNA and RNA synthesis and stopping the growth of cancer cells. Once administered, the drug is concentrated especially on neoplastic tissue. Fluorouracil is used to treat several types of cancer including colon, rectum and head and neck cancers. It is also used for other types of cancer, and the skin cream is used for other conditions as well as skin neoplasms and precancerous lesions, such as actinic keratosis, and also for non-malignant lesions as genital warts. Commonly, Fluorouracil can cause side effects such as low platelet and white blood cell count, darkening of skin and nail beds, nausea and vomiting, poor appetite, sores in mouth, lips, or throat, hair loss or thinning, diarrhea, brittle nails, increased sensitivity to sun, dry, flaky and cracking skin. Less commonly, it can raise darkening and hardening of veins used for giving the drug, headache, weakness, muscle aches, and rarely can provoke trouble walking, trouble forming words, and poor coordination, irritated eyes, increased tears, watering eyes, blurred vision, heart problems, confusion, tingling, numbness, or swelling in the hands and feet, and severe allergic reaction. Despite those side effects, Fluorouracil is a safe drug for the treatment of cancers cited above.

Chapter V - Sixty-five eyes of 61 consecutive patients with an intraocular pressure (IOP) over 21 mmHg; without bleb or with a thick, flat bleb after the second postoperative week following trabeculectomy were enrolled in the study. Needle revision was performed initially using a 26-gauge tuberculin syringe containing 5 mg (0.2ml) 5-Fluorouracil (5-FU) within a period of two weeks to 6 months postoperatively after unsuccessful digital massage and/or laser suture-lysis. 5-FU injection was not performed when bleb formation was observed during needling. In case of no bleb formation, 5-FU was injected subconjunctivally over the scleral flap area and repeated weekly for a maximum of six times until a functioning bleb was maintained. Needle revision was successful in 18 of 65 eyes (27.7%) as an initial procedure and 12 eyes (18.5%) maintained success. Fifty-three eyes (81.5%) had 5-FU injection since needle revision did not provide bleb formation (47 eyes) or did not maintain initial success (6 eyes). Mean intraocular pressure was 28.2+4.9 mmHg (range: 22-41) before any intervention and decreased to 20.4+4.8 mmHg (range: 10-35) after a mean follow-up of 32.2 months and the difference was statistically significant (p<0.001). Mean IOP after needle revision in 18 eyes was 18.8+4.9 (range: 8-29) and 16.2+3.8 mmHg in twelve out of 18 patients that maintained success. Mean IOP after the last 5-FU injection was 21.2+4.6 mmHg (range: 12-35). The mean number of 5-FU injections was 2.4 (range:1-6). During a mean follow-up of 32.2 months (range: 1-56 months) three eyes (4.6%) had diffuse corneal punctate epitheliopathy lasting for 2-3 weeks and subconjuctival hemorrhage was seen in 10 eyes (15.4%). The drug leaked into the anterior chamber causing no complications in one eye and immediate superior limbal vascularization of the cornea was observed in one eye. Needle revision and/or subconjuctival 5-FU injection over the flap area is a safe and relatively efficient approach with low rate of minor complications in the management of bleb failure in long term as well as in the early postoperative period.

Chapter VI - The dose of chemotherapeutic agents is considered to be a limiting factor in the treatment of cancer. An ideal chemotherapeutic strategy could be to deliver a high concentration of drug that would be released in sustained small amounts from targeted microspheres to effectively kill only tumour cells but yet reduce toxicity to normal tissue. This theory was tested *in vitro* before it was evaluated in a rodent model. We showed that small amounts of drugs were released in a sustained fashion over a two week period. Cells of a rodent ovarian carcinoma cell line were exposed to cisplatin and 5-fluorouracil, either as free drug or encapsulated in albumin microspheres that were either conjugated to monoclonal antibodies or not. Clonogenic and cell survival growth curve assays, as well as micronucleus assays, were used to determine the feasilbility of employing targeted immunomicrospheres as a treatment regimen for ovarian cancer. In cell survival growth curve assays, cell survival was reduced to 1.2% of the control and in clonogenic assays it was reduced to 7.87% when cells were treated with drug-containing immunomicrospheres. 3.2-fold more micronuclei were found in those cells that had been exposed to the drugs in immunomicrospheres than in those subjected to untargeted microspheres. Thus, these results indicate that immunomicrospheres are more effective in delivering cisplatin and 5-fluorouracil directly to the target cells than the unconjugated microspheres. To evaluate this regimen *in vivo*, a DMBA-OC-1R tumour was removed from a Wistar rat and passaged into healthy animals that subsequently developed tumours. 60% of the animals that were treated with 10 mg/kg CDDP and 40 mg/kg 5-FU administered via immunomicrospheres, survived a 90 day time period in comparison to rats treated with 5 mg/kg CDDP and 20 mg/kg 5-FU in its free form. These results suggest that targeted chemotherapy could be an effective option in the treatment of ovarian cancer as high concentrations of chemotherapeutic drugs can be delivered in sustained fashion at the target site with a reduction of systemic cytotoxic side-effects to normal tissue.

In: Fluorouracil
Editors: A. Longinho and S. Dobreiro

ISBN: 978-1-62081-970-8
© 2012 Nova Science Publishers, Inc.

Chapter I

ACYCLIC 5-FLUOROURACIL *O*, *N*-ACETALS: ANTIPROLIFERATIVE ACTIVITIES, CELL-CYCLE REGULATION, APOPTOSIS AND CELLULAR DIFFERENTIATION

Nawal Mahjeb, Angélica Luque, Cayetana Ferrer, Esther Hernández and Joaquín M. Campos[*]

Departamento de Química Farmacéutica y Orgánicam,
Facultad de Farmacia, Granada, Spain

ABSTRACT

The goal of cancer chemotherapy with classical drugs is often complicated by significant toxicity. As an alternative, induced differentiation modulates the cell programme by transforming malignant cells into mature cells with no proliferative potential. Our data demonstrate that (RS)-1-{[3-(2-hydroxyethoxy)-1-*iso*propoxy]propyl}-5-fluorouracil inhibits proliferation, induces myogenic differentiation and increases the expression of proteins specifically present in normally differentiated skeletal muscle cells against the rhabdomyosarcoma cell line RD. From a designing point of view, a benzene ring was fused to the side chain in order to increase the lipophilicity of the molecules. Herein we report the preparation and biological activity of

[*] corresponding author; e-mail: jmcampos@ugr.es; Tel. (+34) 958243850, fax: (+34) 958243845.

three compounds being (*RS*)-1-[2-(5-substituted-2-hydroxybenzyloxy)-1-methoxyethyl]-5-fluorouracils. A catechol-derived compound and two salicyl-derived compounds such as (*RS*)-(*Z*)-1-[4-(2-hydroxyphenyl)-1-methoxy-but-3-enyl]-5-fluorouracil [(*Z*)-**43**] and its dihydrogenated derivative (*RS*)-1-[4-(2-hydroxyphenyl)-1-methoxybutyl]-5-fluorouracil were prepared to complete the set of six *O,N*-acetals. The most active compound against the MCF-7 breast cancer cell line was (*Z*)-**43** (IC$_{50}$ = 9.40 ± 0.64 μM). Differentiated breast cancer cells generate fat deposits within the cytoplasm. The MCF-7 cells treated with (*Z*)-**43** caused an increase in the lipid content over control cells after 3 days of treatment. Our results suggest that there may be significant potential advantages in the use of this new differentiating agent for the treatment of breast cancer.

Keywords: Acyclic *O,N*-Acetals, Acyclonucleosides, Breast cancer, Cellular Differentiation, 5-Fluorouracil

INTRODUCTION

Although 5-fluorouracil (5-FU) was first introduced in 1957, it remains an essential part of the treatment of a wide range of solid tumours. 5-FU has antitumour activity against epithelial malignancies arising in the gastrointestinal tract, breast as well as the head and neck, with single-agent response rates of only 10-30% [1]. As all the anticancer agents, 5-FU leads to several toxicities. Mielotoxicity is the major toxic effect in patients receiving bolus doses. Hand-foot syndrome (palmar-plantar erythrodysesthesia), stomatitis, neuro- and cardiotoxicity are associated with continuous infusions. Other adverse effects associated with both bolus-dose and continuous infusion regimens include nausea and vomiting, diarrhea, alopecia and dermatitis. All these reasons explain the need for more effective and less toxic 5-FU derivatives. Therefore, novel derivatives of 5-FU possessing a broader spectrum of antitumour activity and fewer toxic side effects than 5-FU have been sought diligently in a number of laboratories The emergence of acyclovir, 9-[(2-hydroxyethoxy)methyl]guanine [2] as an excellent antiviral agent has stimulated the synthesis of a wide variety of acyclic nucleosides (or *seco*-nucleosides) modified either in the base moiety or the acyclic part [3]. The antiviral action of these substances or their metabolites is generally due to an inhibition of DNA polymerases. It is known that *Cidofovir*, the cytosine-derived carboacyclic pronucleotide, exhibits potent *in vitro* and *in vivo* activity against a broad spectrum of herpes viruses, including HCMV, and it has been approved for the treatment of HCMV retinitis in AIDS patients [4,5]. 5-(1-

Azidovinyl)-substituted acyclic pyrimidine nucleosides have shown potent anti-HBV activity without significant toxicity [6]. Balzarini *et al.* [7] have recently reported the antiviral activity of acyclic pyrimidine nucleoside phosphonates. New pyrimidine acyclonucleosides are of great interest, with regard to their anticancer activity, since it has been shown that various 5-FU derivatives are active against some malignant cell lines due to an inhibition of thymidylate synthase by the formation of 5-fluorodeoxyuridine monophosphate or by the incorporation of 5-fluorouridine monophosphate into RNA. In some malignant tumours the activity of uridine phosphates is enhanced [8]; therefore, 5-FU acyclonucleosides may even exhibit a higher antitumour activity with simultaneously lower toxicity than 5-FU [8].

In this review we report the synthesis and antitumour activity of the acyclonucleoside 5-FU derivatives **2** through the $SnCl_4$-catalyzed opening of alkoxy-1,4-diheteroepanes **1** (Scheme 1) by 2,4-bis-*O*-trimethylsilyl-5-fluorouracil **3** generated *in situ* in acetonitrile. Acyclonucleosides of type **2** are especially interesting due to the following two reasons (a) the presence of the hydroxyl group in the side chain that could therefore be phosphorylated, and (b) they constitute a new class of antitumour agents, since 5-FU is bound to a cytostatic aldehyde such as acrolein [14] or some of its homologues and, accordingly two active substances are combined in one drug

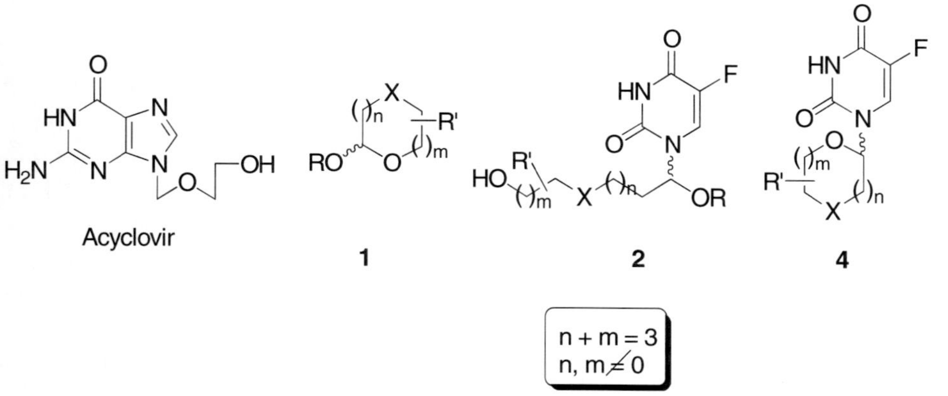

Acyclovir

1

2

4

$$n + m = 3$$
$$n, m \neq 0$$

Scheme 1.

PREPARATION AND BIOLOGICAL ACTIVITY OF 1-{[3-(2-HYDROXYETHYLHETERO)]-1-ALKOXY]PROPYL}-5-FLUOROURACILS 2A-F AND 1-{[2-(3-HYDROXYPROPOXY)]-1-*ISO*PROPOXY]ETHYL}-5-FLUOROURACIL 2G

Chemistry

The reaction of 2,4-bis-*O*-trimethylsilyl-5-fluorouracil **3** (Scheme 2) generated *in situ* [from hexamethyldisilazane (HMDS) and chlorotrimethylsilane (CTS)] with the seven-membered cycloacetals **1** in acetonitrile afforded the desired products **2** after the addition of 1.25 equivalents of tin(IV) chloride. The reaction was completed within 0.5-1.25 h and then quenched by a concentrated aqueous solution of sodium bicarbonate. The products were purified by flash chromatography using chloroform/methanol mixtures.

Table 1 lists reaction times and yields obtained for compounds **2**. The (*RS*)-5-*iso*propoxy-6-methyl-1,4-dioxepane **1d** and the (*RS*)-5-*iso*propoxy-7-methyl-1,4-dioxepane **1e** have been used as the *trans* and *cis* isomers, respectively, and they give rise to the racemic mixture of diastereoisomers **2d** and **2e**, both being pairs of diastereoisomers formed in equal quantities Thus, the title reaction is regiospecific but not diastereoselective It was not possible to separate both diastereoisomers of **2d**. Nevertheless, (1*R**,3*R**)-**2e** and (1*R**,3*S**)-**2e** were separated by flash chromatography although they were tested against HEp human cells as the racemic mixture of both diastereoisomers (Table 1). The present synthetic method is rapid and economical, does not seem to present serious scaling-up problems and is clearly adaptable to the synthesis of other pyrimidine acyclonucleosides [10] for the biological evaluation of their antitumour and/or antiviral properties. It is essential to maintain anhydrous conditions during the transformations; to obtain good yields it is also advisable to work under argon or nitrogen.

The reaction was carried out under several different concentrations of SnCl$_4$ and different temperatures, even as low as -35 °C, and the presence of the cyclic seven-membered structures **4** was not detected.

The regiospecificity outcome observed could be accounted for by the fact that SnCl$_4$ readily forms octahedral complexes with two donor molecules (e.g., ether, THF) or with bidentate ligand systems [11]. The results were consistent with an intermediate of type **5** in which the (*RS*)-alkoxy-1,4-diheteropane **1** was tied up by SnCl$_4$ (Scheme 2). This hypothesis provided the driving force for the cleavage of the endocyclic acetalic C-O to take place giving the oxocarbenium **6** as the only electrophilic acetalic moiety with concomitant formation of $SnCl_4OR^-$. The mild nucleophilic silylated base **3**, which did not destroy chelation was then able to attack the stable cation 6 to afford the opened *O,N*-acetal **2**, in a S_N1-like reaction, The existence of the oxocarbenium **6** was supported by the increased yield on going from (*RS*)-5-methoxy-1,4-dioxepane **1a** (31%) to (*RS*)-5-*iso*propoxy-1,4-dioxepane **1b** (72%) as starting materials, with an increasing α-branching in relation to the oxonium ion of **6**. The approximate obtained 1:1 ratio of the diastereoisomers of **2d** and **2e** also supported the S_N1 character of the title reaction. As a background to the complexation hypothesis, it has been reported that the reaction of silylated bases with oxathiolanyl and dioxolanyl ring systems and cytosine produced only the β isomer [12,13].

The following two factors proved the mechanism proposed: 1) the dependence of chelation on the identity of the non-acetalic heteroatom of the seven-membered ring [10a]. For instance, when X = *N*Me (Scheme 1, formulae **1, 5** and **2**), the reaction proceeded with a very low yield (14%) [10a], probably because the great basicity of the electronic pair of the *N* atom led to a strong *N*-Sn bond. At the same time, its strength caused the weakening of the other anchorage point, *i.e.*, the Sn-acetalic oxygen atom. It therefore seemed that "activation" by the introduction of a strong electron-withdrawing group on the nitrogen atom was required. As the basicity lessened due to the *p*-tosyl group (**5**, X = *N*Ts), the chelate was more balanced and an adequate charge deficiency was produced on the acetalic carbon leading to the oxocarbenium **6** which accordingly, was susceptible to being attacked by **3** (30%) [10a]; and 2) using and acid incapable of chelation, such as $BF_3 \cdot OEt_2$ [14] maintaining the same experimental conditions, including the acid concentration, the experimental results proved to be different, yielding the aminal acrolein derivative **7**, **2b** and its isomer **8**, in which the acyclic chain was linked through C-1 to the *N*-3 of the 5-fluorouracil moiety (Scheme 3).

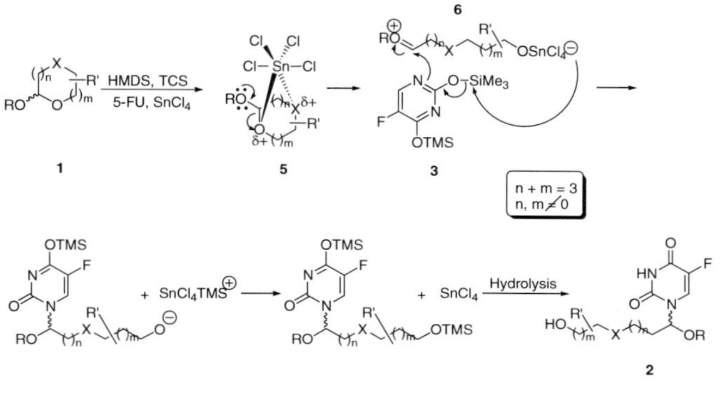

Scheme 2. Proposed mechanism for the formation of acyclonucleosides **2**.

Table 1. Reactions of (*RS*)-alkoxy-1.4-diheteroepanes 1 with 5-FU and biological activities of 2

Comp. No.	Alkoxy-1,4-diheteroepanes 1	Time (h)	Yield (%)	Acyclonucleosides 2	IC_{50}^{a} (µM)
a	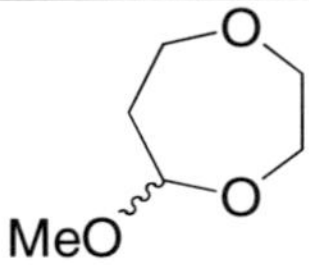 (MeO-substituted 1,4-dioxepane)	0.75	31	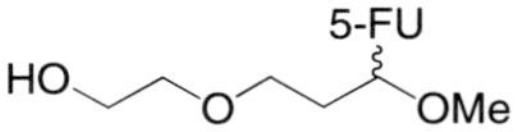 HO—O—(5-FU)—OMe	-
b	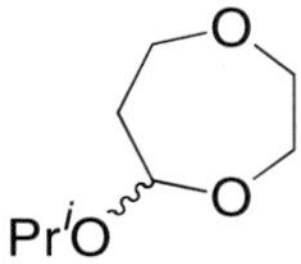 (Pr^iO-substituted 1,4-dioxepane)	0.50	72	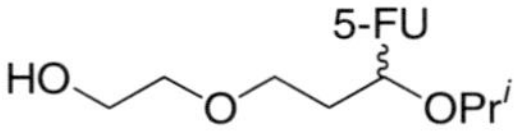 HO—O—(5-FU)—OPr^i	45
c	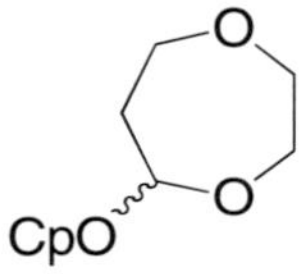 (CpO-substituted 1,4-dioxepane)	0.50	62[b]	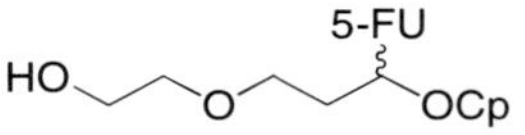 HO—O—(5-FU)—OCp	18
d	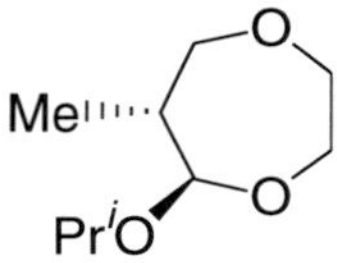 (Me, Pr^iO-substituted 1,4-dioxepane)	0.50	68[c]	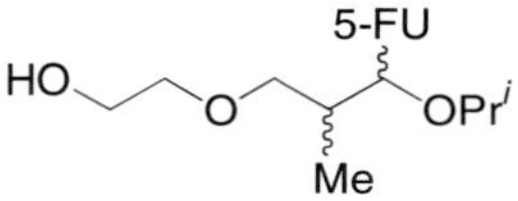 HO—O—(5-FU)—OPr^i, Me	45
e	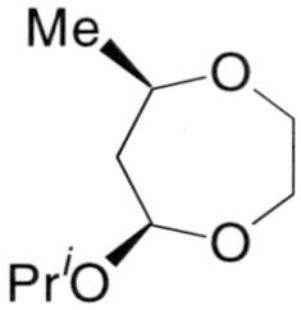 (Me, Pr^iO-substituted 1,4-dioxepane)	1.25	57[d]	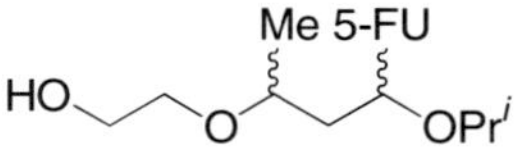 HO—O—(Me, 5-FU)—OPr^i	25
f	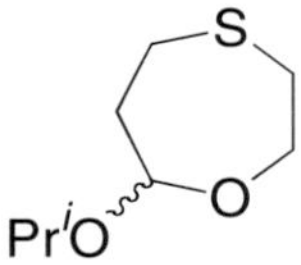 (Pr^iO-substituted 1,4-oxathiepane)	0.75	86	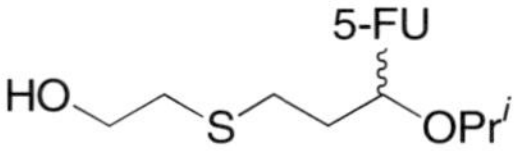 HO—S—(5-FU)—OPr^i	362
g	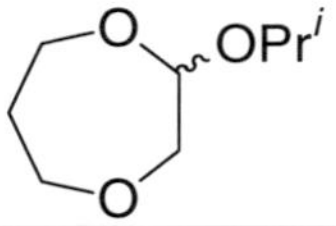 (OPr^i-substituted 1,4-dioxepane)	0.50	70	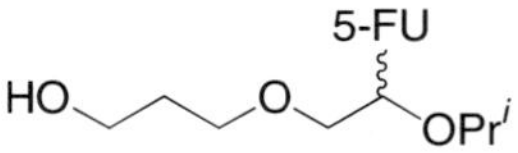 HO—O—(5-FU)—OPr^i	4300

[a] The antitumour activities of compounds **2** were tested against Hep-2 human cells (IC_{50} = 90 µM, 5-FU). IC_{50} is the fifty percent inhibitory concentration, *i.e.* the concentration required to inhibit the growth of treated cells to 50% of untreated controls.

[b] Cp = Cyclopentyl.

[c] (Racemic) diastereomer mixture was not separated.

[d] (Racemic) diastereomer mixture was separated, but was tested as such mixture.

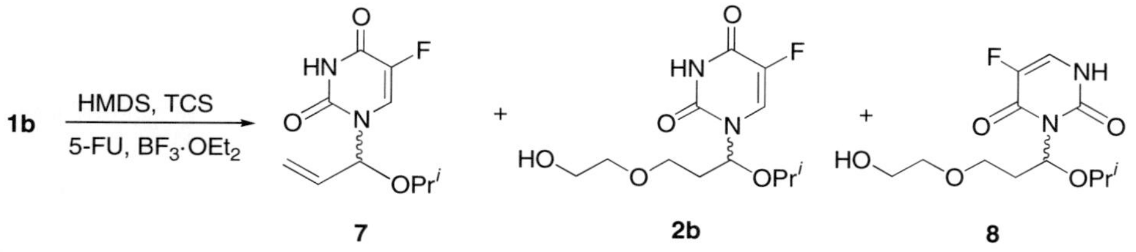

Scheme 3. "Abnormal behaviour" when boron trifluoride etherate is used as Lewis acid.

The global sum of the yields of **7** (14%), **2b** (22.7%) and **8** (28.8%) was roughly the same yield as **2b** (72%, Table 1) obtained by the $SnCl_4$-mediated regioespecific opening of **lb**. The formation of **2b** may be explained by the electrophilic attack of the BF_3 in its etherate form on the endocyclic acetalic oxygen atom of **lb** whereas the more likely explanation for the formation of **7** would involve the BF_3 complex on *O*-1 of **lb** and the one-step proton β-elimination (on the three-carbon moiety) and subsequent leaving of the ethylene glycol moiety. The "rare" 5-FU *N*-3 acyclonucleoside **8** could be rationalized on the basis of "Vorbrüggen's σ-complex" [15] presumably due to prior complexation between the Lewis acid and the *N*-1 atom of the silylated base **3**, assuming the greatest acidity strength of BF_3 against $SnCl_4$ [16a]. Thus, BF_3 shows no advantage over the corresponding reaction with $SnCl_4$. In short, the products obtained using $BF_3 \cdot OEt_2$ are explained through complexation on *O*-1 and *O*-4 of the cycloacetal **lb,** proving that they are more basic than the exocyclic acetalic oxygen whose complexation and subsequent attack of the nucleophile **3** should have yielded the non-detected (*RS*)-1-(1,4-dioxepane-5-yl)-5-fluorouracil.

The starting cycloacetals [17] **la-f** were obtained by acid-catalyzed alcoholysis at room temperature of the dioxolane hydroxyacetals **9-12** (Scheme 4).

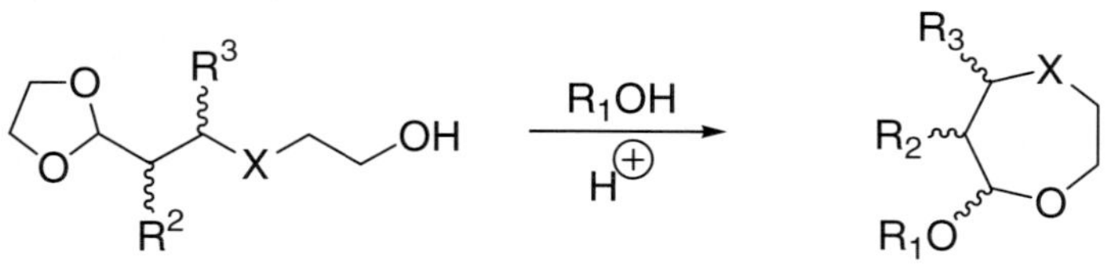

9 $R^2 = R^3 = H$; $X = O$
10 $R^2 = Me$; $R^3 = H$; $X = O$
11 $R^2 = H$; $R^3 = Me$; $X = O$
12 $R^2 = R^3 = H$; $X = S$

1c $R^1 = Cp$; $R^2 = R^3 = H$; $X = O$
1d $R^1 = Pr^i$; $R^2 = Me$; $R^3 = H$; $X = O$
1e $R^1 = Pr^i$; $R^2 = H$; $R^3 = Me$; $X = O$
1f $R^1 = Pr^i$; $R^2 = R^3 = H$; $X = S$

Scheme 4.

(*RS*)-5-Methoxy- and (*RS*)-5-*iso*propoxy-1,4-dioxepanes **la** and **1 b,** respectively, were reported by us [17] and also **9** [17]. Compounds **10** and **11** were prepared in a one-pot reaction between the corresponding α,β-unsaturated aldehydes and ethylene glycol in dichloromethane/hydrochloric acid [17].

The reaction between **10** and *iso*propanol under sulfuric acid catalysis yielded the (*RS*)-*trans*-**ld** isomer [with 7 % of the (*RS*)-*cis* isomer] whereas the same reaction carried out on **11** gave rise to the (*RS*)-*cis*-**le** isomer (with 4% of the (*RS*)-*trans* isomer). In the former case, besides (*RS*)-*trans*-**ld,** 2-(3-*iso*propoxy-2-propyl)-1,3-dioxolane was obtained as a result of a ring contraction of the seven-membered ring. A similar contraction was previously documented in our previous paper [22]. Compound **12** was prepared by the treatment of 3-chloropropanal ethylene acetal with the sodium mercaptide of 2-mercaptoethanol in dry ethanol [17].

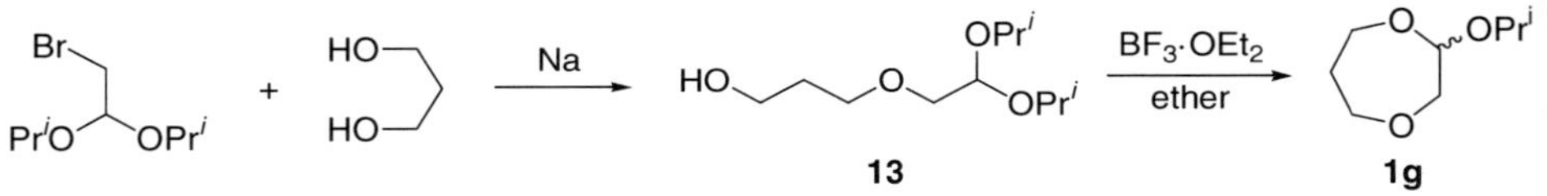

Scheme 5. Synthesis of (*RS*)-2-*iso*propoxy-1,4-dioxepane **1g**.

The synthesis of (*RS*)-2-*iso*propoxy-l,4-dioxepane **lg** was carried out following a similar procedure used for the preparation of 2-methoxy-1,4-dioxepane [18] (Scheme 5).

Biological Activity

In Vitro Antitumour Activity

The antitumour activity of **2b-g** was tested against HEp human cells *in vitro* and the results are shown in Table 1. Generally speaking, it can be said a) that the most active compound ($IC_{50} = 18$ μM) is **2c**, the most lipophilic structure being due to the cyclopentoxy moiety, and b) the less active compound ($IC_{50} = 4300$ μM) is **2g**, which cannot give rise to acrolein [19] by enzymic cleavage of the aminal fragment, under non oxidative conditions.

Toxicity: In Vivo Trials. Method A

The toxicity test (**2f**) was carried out on mice of the Mus Musculus species, Swiss albino race, healthy, of 10-12 cm of length (excluding tail), which reach a weight of 30-35 g when adult. Each mouse was administered single dosages of 50, 100, 200, 500 and 1000 mg/kg of weight to statistically representative animal lots. Mice of an average weight of 26 g were used for the 25-200 dosages. Animal lots of 27 g of average weight were used for the highest dosages of 500 and 1000 mg/kg. The growth of the mice was followed through weight control. Neither signs of short-term nor long-term acute toxicity were assessed since the animals died when their biological cycle finished.

Method B

A control study with commercial 5-FU has been carried out, starting with a group of 10 female OF1 mice, some six weeks old. After weighing them and calculating the average weight in grams (24 g), the daily dose that each of them was to receive was established: 4.8 mg/mouse equivalent of 200 mg/kg, a concentration similar to the LD_{50} of 5-FU (180 mg/kg). Each mouse was inoculated with 0.5 mL of 5-FU in accumulative doses, *i.e.*, from day 0 to day 6. With **2b, 2c, 2d** (diastereomeric mixture) and **2e** (diastereomeric mixture) the same procedure was followed, keeping in mind both the percentage of 5-FU contained in our molecules and the quantity of 5-FU present in the pattern of LD_{50} that was established corresponding to the 200 mg/kg aforementioned. The mice treated with 5-FU clearly showed a daily loss of weight compared with the controls. This loss was accompanied by changes in the aspect of the animals, such as changes in the hair and its loss and irritation of the anal zone. In the same way, a reduction in the vital activity of the individuals treated was observed. On the seventh day and after the last injection of 5-FU, eight of the ten mice treated died and the remaining two died a day later. Comparison of these results with those of the above-mentioned drugs showed obvious differences. As in the controls, the change in weight followed no definite tendency, there was no variation in the aspect of the mice and no signs of apparent toxicity were observed. More conclusively, death did not occur due to each treatment. The animals died when their biological cycle finished.

CHEMICAL MODIFICATIONS ON THE ACYCLIC MOIETY OF 3-(2-HYDROXYETHOXY)-1-ALKOXYPROPYL NUCLEOBASES

Chemistry

The synthesis of the modified acyclonucleosides **14-24** (Table 2) will be shown in this section. The chemical modifications include the irreversible blocking of the hydroxy function (**14** and **15**), substitution of the hydroxy group by the chlorine atom (**16**) or the oxidation to a methoxycarbonyl group (**17**), the increase in lipophilicity (**18-21**, in which the acyclic chain is linked to several nucleobases), the increase in hydrophilicity (**22**), and the inclusion of the chlorohydrin fragment in the two-carbon atom acyclic chain (**23**). The (*RS*)-*bis*(5-fluorouracil-1-yl) compound **24** was also included in this study.

All the structures **14-24** can be seen as prodrugs of the nucleobases, with an acrolein moiety within them. After the expected chemical or enzymatic hydrolysis, two biologically active substances could thus be generated from the same drug as a consequence of drug activation. Acrolein itself inhibits the growth of Chinese hamster ovary cells (IC_{50} = 50 μM) [9]. To test behaviour of the products on cellular systems, cytotoxic activity against the HT-29 colon carcinoma [20] was determined [21], and the most active compound was used to study the modifications in proliferation and degree of differentiation in the human rhabdomyosarcoma cell line RD.

As starting materials for the synthesis of **14**, **15**, **17-21**, and **23**, the acetals **25** [22], **28** [22], and **29** [22] (Table 3) were used, under our standard conditions [17]. These synthetic conditions were also used for the preparation of the adenine (**18** and **19**) and the uracil (**20**) derivatives, respectively. There are two facts that are worth pointing out:

a) The condensation of olefin **28** with adenine in the presence of tin(IV) chloride, HMDS and CTS in anhydrous acetonitrile at room temperature for 19 h proceeded regioselectively: the *N*-7 and *N*-9-acyclonucleosides **18** and **19** (see Table 3) were isolated in 31% and 10% yields, respectively (*N*-7/*N*-9 ratio = 3:1).

Table 2. Structures of the modified acyclonucleosides 14-24

$$Y\diagdown X \diagdown\diagup\diagdown OR$$

Base

Comp.	R	X	Y	Base
14	Me	O	CH$_2$OTs	5-FU
15	Me	S	CH$_2$OMe	5-FU
16	Me	O	CH$_2$Cl	5-FU
17	Me	O	COOMe	5-FU
18	Pr^i	O	CH=CH$_2$	Ad-7-yl[a]
19	Pr^i	O	CH=CH$_2$	Ad-9-yl[a]
20	Pr^i	O	CH=CH$_2$	U
21	Pr^i	O	CH=CH$_2$	5-FU
22	Pr^i	O	CH(OH)CH$_2$OH	5-FU
23	Me	O	CH(OH)CH$_2$Cl	5-FU
24	Me	O	CH(OMe)5-FU	5-FU

[a]Ad = Adenine

When tin(IV) chloride was replaced by trimethylsilyl trifluoromethanesulfonate, the reaction led to the formation of the *N*-9-acyclonucleoside **19** as the principal product (50 %) along with the formation of the *N*-7-acyclonucleoside **18** in 26 % yield (*N*-7/*N*-9 ratio ≈ 1:2) [23]. The Lewis acid should generally be strong enough to convert derivatives into their corresponding oxocarbenium ions (such as **6**, Scheme 2). Any additional acidic strength of the Lewis acid will only result in increased σ-complex formation with the silylated base, which in turn might lead to complications in regioselectivity or reaction rates [24].

As the ^{1}H NMR spectra of **18** and **19** were very similar, the position of the acyclic substituent at the adenine base had to be deduced mainly from the ^{13}C NMR spectra (Table 4).

The site of the adenine aminal C-N bond was determined by comparison of the ^{13}C NMR spectra of the corresponding compounds with those of related adenine *N*-7- and *N*-9-glycosides and *N*-7 and *N*-9-methyl adenine derivatives [25]. The variation of ^{13}C NMR chemical shifts (**18-19**, Δδ in ppm) was calculated when the site of substitution for the 3-allyloxy-l-isopropoxy-l-propyl moiety changed from *N*-7 to *N*-9 in adenine. When the site of attachment of the acyclic moiety is changed from *N*-7 (**18**) to *N*-9 (**19**), one would expect a downfield shift of the C-4 signal approximately equivalent to an upfield shift on the C-5 resonance by analogy with the data obtained for adenine *N*-7 and *N*-9-glycosides and *N*-7 and *N*-9-methyl adenine derivatives [25]. In agreement with these data were the assignments for **18** which denoted a downfield shift of 11.5 ppm for the C-4$_{Ad}$ signal when compared with its position in **19** and an upfield shift of -9.39 ppm for the C-5$_{Ad}$ line. The C-6$_{Ad}$ resonance moved upfield -4.24 ppm because of a steric interaction between the acydic moiety and the amino group and subsequent charge compression in the H_2N-C bond. The C-8$_{Ad}$ resonance position moved downfield 5.52 ppm while the C-2$_{Ad}$ resonance position was practically insensitive to the site of alkylation on the heterocyclic moiety (*N*-7 or *N*-9). The ^{13}C-^{1}H correlation spectra of **18** and **19** unambiguously allowed us to distinguish between H-2$_{Ad}$ (8.47 ppm for **18** and 8.45 ppm for **19**) and H-8$_{Ad}$ (δ 8.00 ppm for **19** and δ 7.98 ppm for **18**). The assignment of the other signals was straightforward. The fact that it is not necessary to protect the amino group of the adenine and the possibility of synthesizing non-naturally-occurring *N*-7- and *N*-9 adenine acyclonucleoside analogues makes this new simplified preparation of particular value especially when these targets have to be prepared quickly.

Table 3. Structures and yields of the modified acyclonucleosides 14, 15, 17, 18, 20, 21 and 23

Acetal	Y	R	Base	Product	Yield (%)
25	CH_2OTs	Me	5-FU	14	68
26	CH_2OMe	Me	5-FU	15	68
27	COOMe	Me	5-FU	17	95
28	$CH=CH_2$	Pr^i	Ad-7-yl	18	31[a]
28	$CH=CH_2$	Pr^i	U	20	30
28	$CH=CH_2$	Pr^i	5-FU	21	72
29	$CH(OH)CH_2Cl$	Me	5-FU	23	58

[a]Ad = Adenine. Compound **19** (Ad-9-yl derivative) was also obtained in 10% yield.

Table 4. ^{13}C NMR chemical shifts[a] (δ, ppm) for the adenine[b] moiety in 18 (*N*-7) and 19 (*N*-9) for $CDCl_3$ solutions

Compound	C-2	C-4	C-5	C-6	C-8
18	153.64	161.64	110.25	151.33	144.22
19	153.27	150.14	119.64	155.57	138.70

[a]Each reading was quoted to the nearest 0.05 ppm.
[b]The locants correspond to the IUPAC enumeration of adenine.

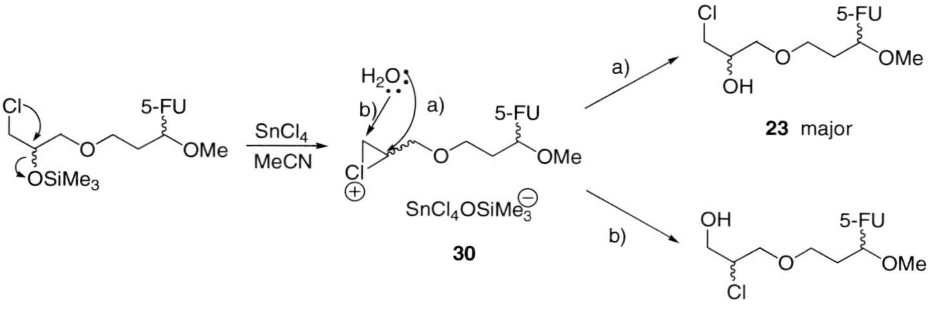

Scheme 6.

b) The reaction of **29** with 5-FU under standard conditions [22] led to acyclonucleoside **23**. In addition to **23**, a very minor close-moving spot was also separated by careful chromatography on silica gel (CHCl$_3$/MeOH: 100/3) whose ^{1}H (300 MHz) and ^{13}C NMR (75 MHz) data showed to be a mixture of diastereoisomers (Scheme 6).

Their mass spectrum showed the molecular ion at 310, corresponding to a 3:1 doublet due to the chlorine. All these data were consistent with the primary alcohol-bearing acynucleoside **31** formed through the chloronium ion **30** as depicted in Scheme 6. Chlorine is a very weak neighbouring group and can be shown to act in this way only when the solvent does not interfere [16b]. Compound **23** (as a mixture of diastereoisomers) turned out to be the only active compound against HT-29 cells (*vide infra*). All the attempts to separate both diastereoisomers were fruitless. Compounds **16** and **22** (as a mixture of diastereoisomers) had to be prepared from the corresponding acyclonucleosides **32** and **21**, respectively, by using a mixture of PPh$_3$ and CCl$_4$ and DMF as a solvent, and by hydroxylation of the exocyclic double bond on treatment with osmium tetroxide and *N*-methylmorpholine *N*-oxide (NMO) in aqueous acetone, respectively (Scheme 7). It was previously reported [26] that 3-(2-hydroxyethoxy)propanal dimethyl acetal cyclized to (*RS*)-5-methoxy-1,4-dioxepane when treated with the Ph$_3$P/CCl$_4$ system, not yielding the expected 3-(2-chloroethoxy)propanal dimethyl acetal, which had to be the synthon for the one-pot preparation of **16**. On the other hand, 3-(2,3-dihydroxypropoxy)propanal dimethyl acetal, obtained by hydroxylation of 3-allyloxypropanal dimethyl acetal in 56% yield, failed in its condensation with 5-FU using SnCl$_4$, probably due to its instability in the acidic medium.

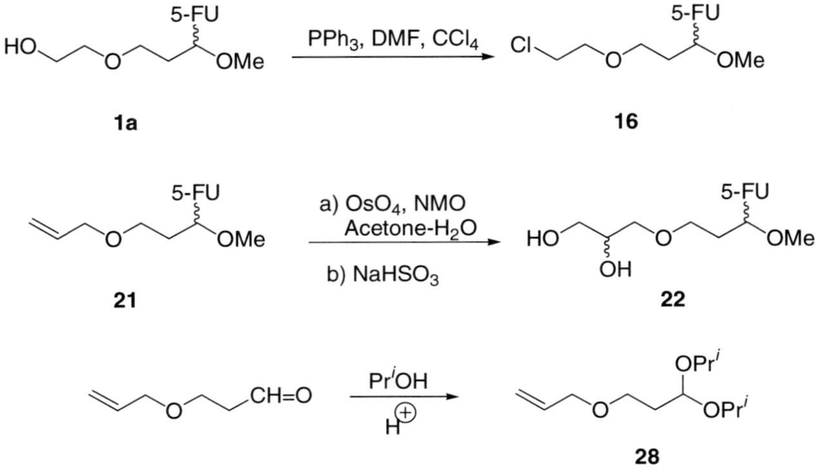

Scheme 7.

Acetal **28** was obtained by acid-catalyzed acetalization of 3-allyloxypropanal [27] with anhydrous/*iso*propanol in 50% yield (Scheme 7). Hydroxyacetal **32** [22] was the starting material that led to the tosyloxy acetal **33**, and to the modified acyclonucleosides **17** and **24** as depicted in Scheme 8.

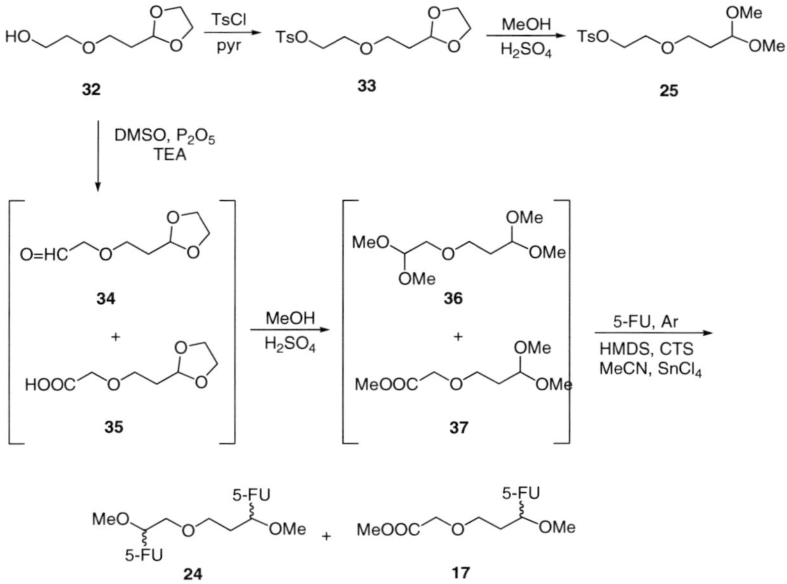

Scheme 8.

When **32** was subjected to dimethyl sulfoxide (DMSO) and P_2O_5-Et_3N (TEA) conditions [28] in the hope of obtaining the aldehyde **34**, the chemical and spectroscopic behaviour of the reaction mixture showed us the presence of another substance, which proved to be the carboxylic acid **35**, formed under the very mild conditions used [29]. As it was not possible to separate both compounds (**34** and **35**) using flash chromatography or distillation under diminished pressure, the synthetic route was continued in the hope that the mono(5-fluorouracil-1-yl) derivative **17** and the bis(5-fluorouracil-1-yl) derivative **24** would be separated by flash chromatography, due to their different lipophilicities. In fact, our assumptions proved to be correct and **17** and **24** were isolated by flash chromatography. The fact that on the one hand, two substances (**34** and **35**) were formed in the reaction, and on the other, the inability to separate them, might be overlooked because of its limited or null chemical synthetic value. But the failure in the oxidation of the primary alcohol of **32** to a formyl group using pyridinium chlorochromate [30], pyridinium dichromate [31] or to a carboxylic acid group by potassium permanganate/18-crown-6 [32], or the Jones reagent [33] circumvented the above drawbacks and made the aforementioned procedure useful, especially when the two final products **17** and **24** were finally separated and isolated. Another approach such as the two possible Williamson syntheses, *i.e.,* from methyl hydroxyacetate and 2-(2-bromoethyl)-1,3-dioxolane, or methyl bromoacetate and 2-(2-hydroxyethyl)-1,3-dioxolane (unpublished results), also failed or gave exceedingly low yields and so prevented the production of usable quantities of material to proceed further in the following steps of the convergent synthesis of **17**.

Biological Activity

Considerable evidence indicates that the malignant phenotype in cancers is not an irreversible state, but represents a disease of altered maturation. Recent years have seen the development of the concept of differentiation therapy based on the conversion of malignant cells to a more benign phenotype through induced differentiation using chemical substances [34]. Research has shown that rhabdomyosarcoma cells can be induced to a differentiated stage with no proliferative potential by antineoplastic drugs such as cytarabine [35] and the antibiotic actinomycin D [36]. Rhabdomyosarcomas are the most common malignant soft-tissue tumours in children comprising 5 % of all pediatric malignances [37]. The degree of rhabdomyosarcoma cell differentiation has been determined by the classic marker desmin [38]; more recently α-actinin and tropomyosin expression have also been used to determine the degree of cytoskeletal organization [39].

In Vitro Cytotoxicily Versus HT-29

The cytotoxic activity of **14-18**, and **20-24** was assessed with the 3-(4,5-dimethylthiazol-2-yl)-2,5-diphenyltetrazolium bromide assay against the HT-29 human colon cancer cell line, as described [21]. The only active compound turned out to be **23** (IC_{50} = 70 µM), which is 8-fold less active than 5-fluorouracil (9 µM [44]), the rest of the series showing IC_{50} values greater than 100 µM (insufficient activity up to this concentration to determine IC_{50}).

In Vitro Differentiation and Growth Inhibition in the RD Cell Line

The rhabdomyosarcoma cell line (RD) was obtained from the American Type Culture Collection. Cell culture and preparation of cells for Fluorescence Activated Cell Sorting (FACScan [41]) were as described previously [42]. Four replicate culture flasks (75 cm^2) with 2×10^6 cells each were exposed to a 90 µM solution of **23** together with controls. Cells were induced with **23** until the sixth day, on which the cells corresponding to the treatment of each day were collected.

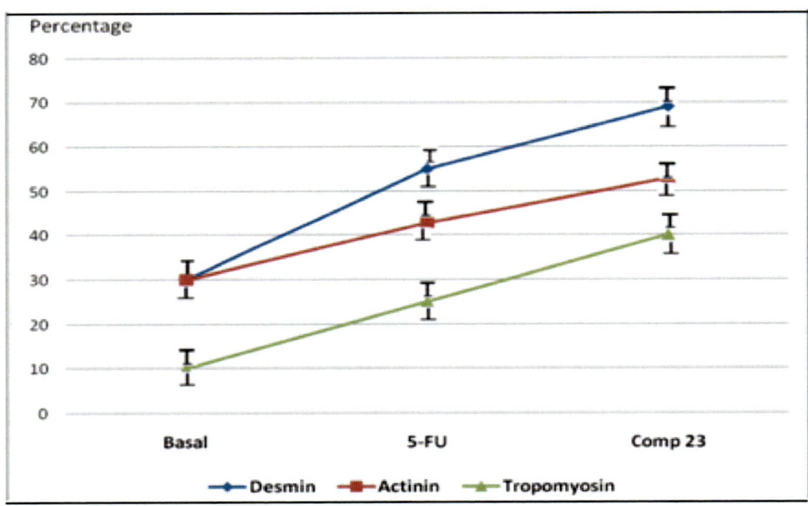

Figure 1. Analysis by fluorescence-activated cell sorting (FACScan). The results are expressed as the percentage of fluorescence corresponding to desmin, α-actinin and tropomyosine expression in RD parental cell line (basal) and RD cells treated with 5-FU (90 µM) and **23** (90 µM).

Quantitative data on the changes in expression of desmin, α-actinin and tropomyosin in RD cell line in RD parental cell line (control), after 6 days of treatment with 5-FU (90 μM), and after 6 days of treatment with **23** (90 μM) were provided by FACS analysis (Figure 1). 5-FU led to clear differentiation signs in the RD cell line. This action has also been demonstrated in the colon carcinoma HT-29 cell line [43]. Nevertheless, 5-FU showed a high cellular toxicity [44] and it was used in short treatments, after which cells were induced to differentiate by classic inductor agents [44b]. Such a differentiative response might imply an important morbidity on healthy tissues. So, the use of **23** presents advantages over 5-FU, *i.e.* a) it is less toxic than 5-FU [22] and b) because it gives rise to a significant increase in the differentiation markers in relation to 5-FU (Figure 1). The inverse relation observed between proliferation and differentiation in tumour and normal cells suggests an alternative approach to cancer therapy that does not involve cell killing, but instead induces malignant cells to differentiate to benign forms with no proliferative potential.

(*RS*)-1-[2-(2-Hydroxymethylphenoxy)-1-Methoxyethyl]-5-Fluorouracils 40b-g: Antiproliferative Activity, Cell Cycle Dysregulation and Apoptotic Induction against Breast Cancer Cells

Breast cancer follows closely on lung cancer as the second leading cancer in women, and is the leading cause of cancer death among women in the 35–54 age group and the second cause of cancer death for women aged 55–74 [45a-c]. The disseminated nature of breast cancer and the development of cross-resistant tumours are the primary causes of failure of current therapies. By the time a tumour is detected, there is a high probability that methastatic lesions will be present, and many of these will already contain a resistant subpopulation of cells. Not surprisingly, there is a substantial interest in the identification of novel anticancer agents for the treatment of breast cancer [45]. Apoptosis or programmed cell death is an innate mechanism by which unwanted, defective, or damaged cells are rapidly and selectively eliminated from the body. It occurs during tissue remodelling, embryonic development, and immune regulation [46]. Apoptosis is the principle mechanism employed by the immune system and chemotherapeutic drugs in eradicating tumour cells. Resistant tumour cells evade the action of anticancer agents by increasing their apoptotic threshold. This has spurred the development of novel chemical compounds capable of inducing apoptosis in chemo/immune-resistant tumour cells. Although breast cancer is most often treated with conventional cytotoxic agents it has proven difficult to induce apoptosis in breast cancer cells using these drugs [47]. By identifying therapies that are particularly effective in activating apoptosis, improved clinical responses may be obtained. Herein the preparation of the acyclic 5-FU *O,N*-acetalic analogues is reviewed, to assess their biological activities against the breast cancer cells.

Chemistry

The synthesis of the *O,N*-acetals was carried out in a two step process: (a) preparation of the intermediate acyclic *O,O*-acetals **38a–f**, and (b) reaction of these acyclic compounds with the pyrimidine base to give the title structures. 5-Chloro-2-hydroxybenzyl alcohols were obtained by reduction of the corresponding salicylaldehyde [48]. Hydroxyacetals **38d–f** were prepared in a similar way to the preparation of **38a–c** [49] by alkylation of the salicyl alcohols (Scheme 9) with bromoacetaldehyde dimethyl acetal, using sodium hydride as a base in anhydrous dimethylformamide (DMF). The substitution of the acetalic OMe group by the 5-FU moiety in the *O,O*-acetals **38a–f** was carried out by reaction with 5-FU in the presence of HMDS and TCS, under acid catalysis of stannic chloride. The aminalic bond is established through *N*-1 of the 5-FU moiety unless otherwise stated.

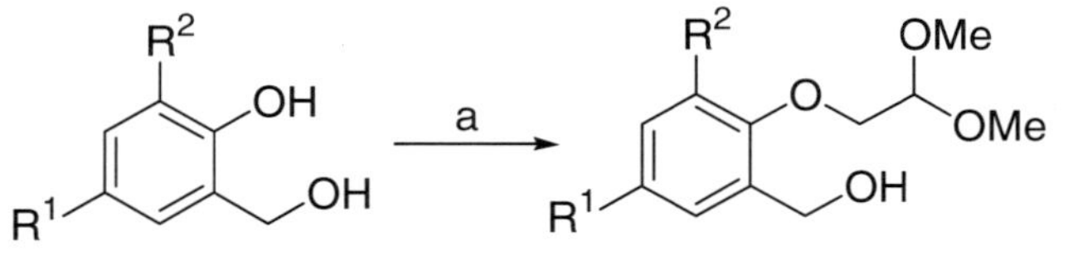

38

a $R^1 = R^2 = H$
b $R^1 = OMe$; $R^2 = H$
c $R^1 = H$; $R^2 = OMe$
d $R^1 = Cl$; $R^2 = H$
e $R^1 = Br$; $R^2 = H$
f $R^1 = NO_2$; $R^2 = H$

Scheme 9. Reagents: (a) $BrCH_2CH(OMe)_2$, NaH, anhydrous DMF.

Table 5. Formation of cyclic and acyclic 5-FU *O,N*-acetals starting from the acyclic *O,O*-acetals 38, the reaction time being 24 h.[a]

Entry	Starting acetal	R^1	R^2	Yield (%) of **39**	Yield (%) of **40**
1	**38b**	OMe	H	26 (5)[b]	27
2	**38c**	H	OMe	-	37
3	**38d**	Cl	H	-	17
4	**38e**	Br	H	-	4 (8)[b]
5	**38f**	NO_2	H	-	35

[a]5-FU, HMDS, TCS, $SnCl_4/CH_2Cl_2$, MeCN.

[b]All the yields refer to compounds in which the 5-FU moiety is linked through *N*-1, except in **40e**[N-3] and **39b**[N-3], in which the link is through *N*-3 and whose yields are reported between brackets.

The condensation between the acyclic *O,O*-acetals **38** and 5-FU gave rise to the cyclic **39** and/or the acyclic *O,N*-acetals **40**, respectively through a process whose regioselectivity depended on the presence and nature of the substituents on the benzene ring (Table 5), named R^1 and R^2. In general, in the majority of cases the attachment of the 5-FU moiety occurred at *N*-1, and rarely at the *N*-3 position of the uracil ring. These facts were confirmed through ^{1}H NMR data. According to Ozaki *et al.* [50] the H-6 coupling pattern of the pyrimidine ring is indicative of the substitution model on the 5-FU moiety. Briefly, (a) a doublet due to C_6-H at around δ 7–8 ppm indicates that 5-FU has a substituent at its *N*-1 position, and (b) a broad triplet due to C_6-H at around δ 7–8 ppm indicates that 5-FU is 3-substituted. Compound **39b**[N-3] (this nomenclature indicates that the 5-FU moiety is linked to the carbon chain through its *N*-3 atom) showed a normal behaviour when the ^{1}H NMR spectrum was recorded in a DMSO-d_6 solution. Nevertheless, the situation is different for **40e**[N-3]: C_6-H resonated as a sharp doublet when the spectrum was recorded in CD_3OD due the rapid exchange of the hydrogen atom of the N_1-H group with the deuterium atom of the solvent. Nevertheless, the aspect of the H-1' casts light on the subject: this proton resonates as a pseudotriplet whereas the same proton of **40e** resonates as a doublet of triplets [δ 5.94 (dt, 1H, H-1', *J*=1.6, 4.0 Hz)], the latter being due to the long-range coupling with the fluoro atom [53], which showed unambiguously that the 5-FU is linked through N-1 to the o-(hydroxymethyl)phenoxyethyl-1-methoxy moiety. In the former case (**40e**$^{N\text{-}3}$), the long-range coupling with the F atom was not observed because its electronic effect was not transmitted through the carbonyl group at position 4 of the uracil ring. In relation with the condensation reaction between the acyclic O,O-acetals **38** and 5-FU, the following can be stated (Table 5):

[1] The nature and position of substituents R^1 and R^2 showed clear influence on both the yields and regioselectivity of the process. Thus, the substitution in position 5 of **38** affected in the following manner (only R^2 = H is considered):

1.1. The electron-withdrawing substituents (Cl, Br and NO_2) induced the preferential formation of acyclic O,N-acetals **40** (entries 3–5).
1.2. The OMe group, the only electron-donating substituent used, halted the regioselectivity of the reaction forming both the cyclic **39** and acyclic **40** O,N-acetals and, moreover, in an approximately 1/1 ratio (entry 1).
1.3. In some cases the presence of substituents in one or other type of O,O-acetals permitted the isolation of derivatives in which the 5-FU moiety was linked through N-3 of the pyrimidine base (entries 1 and 4).

[2] Finally, the substitution in C-3 of **38** by the only group studied (OMe) clearly favoured the formation of the acyclic O,N-acetal (entry 2).

The nitro group of **40f** has been reduced with tin(II) chloride dihydrate in refluxing ethanol to yield **40g** (Scheme 10).

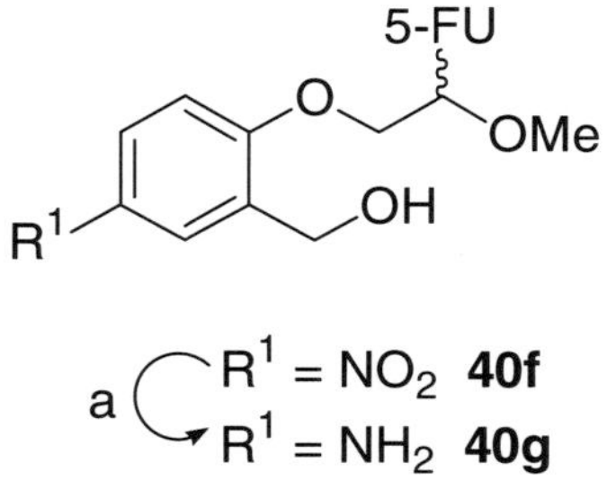

Scheme 10. Reagents: (a) $SnCl_2 \cdot 2H_2O$, EtOH.

BIOLOGICAL ACTIVITIES AGAINST THE HUMAN BREAST CANCER MCF-7

Cell Line

The IC_{50} values of compounds are shown in Table 6. The most active compound is **40f** (5.42 ± 0.26 μM), with an antiproliferative activitiy in the same order as that of Ftorafur (3 ± 0.11 μM). Cell cycle regulation has attracted a great deal of attention as a promising target for cancer research and treatment [51]. The use of cell-cycle-specific treatments in cancer therapy has greatly benefited from the major advances that have been recently made in the identification of the molecular actors regulating the cell cycle and from the better understanding of the connections between cell cycle and apoptosis. As more and more 'cell cycle drugs' are being discovered, their use as anticancer drugs is being extensively investigated [51b]. To study the mechanisms of the antitumour and antiproliferative activities of the compounds, the effects on the cell cycle distribution were analyzed by flow cytometry. DMSO-treated cell cultures contained 68.39% G_0/G_1-phase cells, 12.04% G_2/M-phase cells and 19.57% S-phase cells. In contrast, MCF-7 cells treated during 48 h with the IC_{50} concentrations of **40a,c–g** showed important differences in cell cycle progression compared with DMSO-treated control cells. The treatment with Ftorafur showed a decrease of the G_0/G_1-phase cells and a corresponding accumulation of S-phase cells (45.62% G_0/G_1-phase cells and 54.38% S-phase cells). Moreover, there was an almost total disappearance in the G_2/M population of the cells treated with this drug. In general the cell cycle regulatory activities for the newly synthesized compounds can be divided into the following three groups: (a) compounds **40d** and **40e** accumulated the cancerous cells in the G_2/M-phase, in the former compound at the expense of the S-phase cells, and (b) compound **40f** induced a S-phase cell cycle arrest (50.24%) in a similar percentage to that caused by Ftorafur (54.28%, Table 6). Therefore, it can be affirmed that the nitro derivative (**40f**) may act as a 5-FU prodrug. Nevertheless, this hypothesis needs to be corroborated by further assays. In response to **40a**, the percentage of apoptotic cells increased, from 1.24% in control cells to a maximum of 59.9% apoptotic cells (24 h) at a concentration equal to its IC_{50} against the MCF-7 cell line. This is a remarkable property because the demonstration of apoptosis in MCF-7 breast cancer cells by known apoptosis-inducing agents has proved to be difficult and only few cytotoxic agents act preferentially through an apoptotic mechanism in human breast cancer cells [47,52]. Finally, a fact worth emphasizing is that **40f** (the only compound tested) induced neither toxicity nor death in mice after one month's treatment when administered intravenously twice a week, with a 50 mg/kg dose each time (results not shown).

Table 6. Antiproliferative activities, cell cycle dysregulation, and apoptosis induction in the MCF-7 human breast cancer cell line after treatment for 24 and 48 h for the compounds

Compound	IC_{50} (μM)	Cell cycle (48 h)			Apoptosis (h)	
		G_0/G_1	G_2/M	S	24	48
Control		68.39	12.04	19.57	1.24	1.24
5-FU						
Ftorafur	3 ± 0.11	45.62	0	54.38	52.20	58.06
40a	18.5 ± 0.95	67.18	4.67	28.16	59.90	40.23
40c	29.0 ± 1.63	62.72	1.59	35.69	33.35	37.87
40d	18.0 ± 0.85	71.01	28.99	0.00	44.36	50.64
40e	16.0 ± 1.18	51.45	20.66	27.88	42.24	36.37
40f	5.42 ± 0.26	46.92	2.84	50.24	40.73	48.22
40g	21.0 ± 1.02	67.32	9.40	23.28	41.15	37.81

(*RS*)-1-[2-(2-HYDROXYBENZYLOXY)-1-METHOXYETHYL]-5-FLUOROURACILS 41A-E AND CATECHOL-DERIVED ACYCLIC 5-FU *O,N*-ACETALS 42, (*Z*)-43 AND 44

Chemistry

Molecules **40** [53] are characterized by the presence of ethereal phenoxy and hydroxymethyl groups in an *ortho* relationship. In this section is reviewed the preparation and biological activity of regioisomers of **40**, *i.e.*, compounds characterized by the presence of a free phenolic group and an ethereal methyloxy moiety, having the general formula (*RS*)-1-[2-(5-substituted-2-hydroxybenzyloxy)-1-methoxyethyl]-5-fluorouracils (**41a,d,e**, Scheme 11), (*RS*)-1-[3-(2-hydroxyphenoxy)-1-methoxypropyl]-5-fluorouracil (**42**), (*RS*)-(*Z*)-1-[4-(2-hydroxyphenyl)-1-methoxy-but-3-enyl]-5-fluorouracil (**43**) and its dihydrogenated derivative (*RS*)-1-[4-(2-hydroxyphenyl)-1-methoxybutyl]-5-fluorouracil (**44**, Scheme 11).

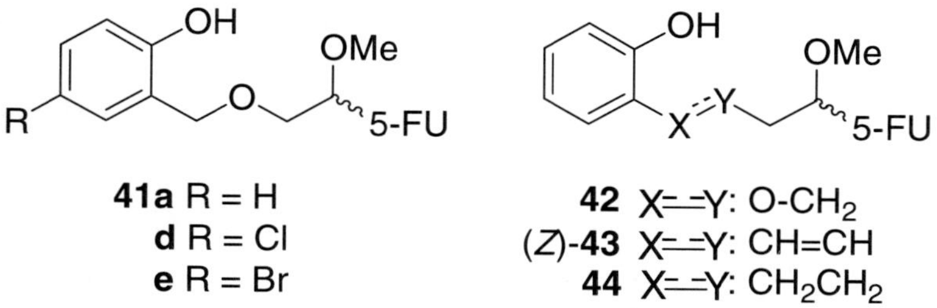

Scheme 11. In all cases the attachment of the 5-FU moiety occurs at the *N*-1 atom of the uracil ring.

The synthesis of derivatives **41a,d,e** was undertaken by previously protecting the phenolic group with the 2-methoxyethoxymethyl (MEM) group to produce compounds **45a,d,e** [54]. Once blocked, the alcoholic group was alkylated with bromoacetaldehyde dimethyl acetal [54], and then the substitution of the OMe group by the 5-FU moiety with the concomitant deblocking of the protecting group was accomplished in a one step/one pot reaction (Scheme 12).

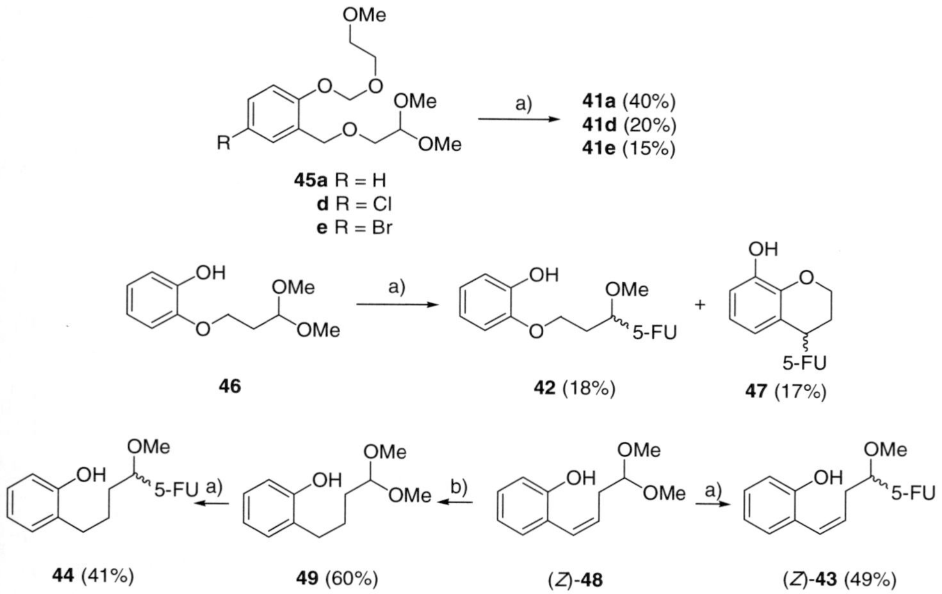

Scheme 12. Reagents: (a) 5-FU, HMDS, TCS, $SnCl_4/CH_2Cl_2$, MeCN; (b) H_2, Pd/C, 4.3 atm, 30 min.

The substitution of the acetalic methoxy group by the 5-FU moiety was carried out in the presence of HMDS and TCS, under acid catalysis (SnCl$_4$) in dry acetonitrile for 24 h. A catechol-derived compound such as (*RS*)-1-[3-(2-hydroxyphenoxy)-1-methoxypropyl]-5-fluorouracil (**42**) and two salicyl-derived compounds such as (*RS*)-(*Z*)-1-[4-(2-hydroxyphenyl)-1-methoxy-but-3-enyl]-5-fluorouracil [(*Z*)-**43**] and its dihydrogenated derivative (*RS*)-1-[4-(2-hydroxyphenyl)-1-methoxybutyl]-5-fluorouracil (**44**) were prepared to complete the set of six acyclic *O,N*-acetals (Scheme 12). It has to be pointed out that the condensation reaction between **46** and 5-FU led to the expected acyclic *O,N*-acetal **42**, in addition to the unexpected six-membered 5-FU derivative **47**, in a ratio of 1 to 1.

We have previously reported the regiospecific formation of **47** (44%) when starting from 4-methoxychroman-8-ol [49]. A possible explanation for the formation of **42** and **47** is the following (Scheme 13):

The Lewis acid SnCl$_4$ favoured the formation of the intermediate **51** after complexation on one of the acetalic OMe groups. Then a nucleophilic attack from 2,4-bis-*O*-trimethylsilyl-5-fluorouracil **3** took place on **51** to produce **52** in a fast step. From here, two processes competed and two alternative routes might be followed:

a) The aqueous workup gave rise to the acyclic *O,N*-acetal **42**.

b) Intermediate **52** might suffer an intramolecular cyclization through the iminium ion intermediate **53**. In this process, the electronic density of the unsubstituted aromatic carbon atom, adjacent to the ethereal oxygen atom, was determinant and favoured by the ethereal oxygen atom of the alkyl chain. Finally, after hydrolysis compound **47** was formed. A similar iminium ion was hypothesized by Hager and Liotta [55] during the formation of the β-anomer of AZT from a non-carbohydrate precursor.

Compound (*Z*)-**48** was reported by us [49]. Its catalytic hydrogenation under 10% Pd/C gave rise to **49**. The corresponding condensation reactions produced (*Z*)-**43** (49%) and **44** (41%) respectively.

It was previously reported that the acidity of phenolic compounds is modulated by electronic effects. *ortho* and *para* electron-releasing groups decrease acidity in relation to the phenol group, whilst electron-withdrawing groups at the same position act in the opposite manner. As a result of both resonance and field/inductive effects, charge concentration led to lesser stability of phenoxy anions and to a decrease in acidity [16c]. Accordingly, the electronic properties of the *ortho* and *para* substituents to the hydroxyl phenoxy group modified the selectivity of the alkylation site by 2-methoxyethoxymethyl chloride (MEMCl) [58]. Due to these reasons, compounds **41b,c** were not obtained and their regioisomers **40b,c** were synthesized instead (Scheme 14).

It is worth pointing out at that **40b** was obtained with the highest yield (26%) [57] when the starting *O,O*-acetal was **38b**, and not the MEM-containing *O,O*-acetal **55b** (8%). Nevertheless, **40c** was obtained approximately with the same yield, regardless of the nature of the starting *O,O*-acetals (40% from **55c**, and 37% from **38c** [53]).

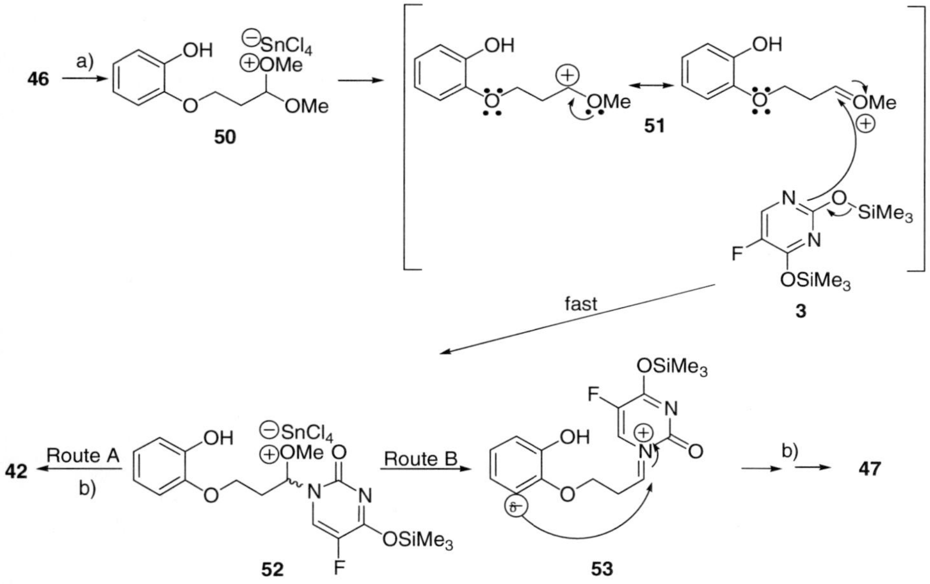

Scheme 13. Reaction mechanism between **46** and 5-FU. Reagents: (a) 5-FU, HMDS, TCS, SnCl$_4$/CH$_2$Cl$_2$, MeCN; (b) H$_2$O.

Biological Results

The anticancer activity of the 5-FU acyclic *O,N*-acetals are shown in Table 7 (entries 5-10). This Table shows the biological activities of **40a**, **40d** and **40e** [64] also, in order to establish the primary structure-activity studies related with the regioisomerism of the compounds.

Structure **40a** (Table 7, entry 2) was $\approx$ 2.4-fold more active than its regioisomer **41a** (Table 7, entry 5). Nevertheless, each pair of the regioisomers **40d** (Table 7, entry 3) and **41d** (Table 7, entry 6), and **40e** (Table 7, entry 4) and

41e (Table 7, entry 7) were equipotent. Taking **40a** as a lead, the strategy of the functional CH_2-O inversion (O-CH_2) was applied and consequently the antiproliferative activity of **42** was measured: compound **42** (Table 7, entry 8) was slightly less active than **40a** (Table 7, entry 2). Next, the exchange of the ether group and the methylene group was undertaken to produce **44**.

From Table 7, entry 10, it seemed that the absence of the ethereal oxygen atom in the side chain was not detrimental to the antiproliferative activity (compare the data of entry 5 with that of entry 10). In order to improve the anticancer activity of **44**, (Z)-**43** was designed and synthesized with the objective to produce an analogue in which the side chain was conformationally restricted around the C-3'-C-4' bond by the presence of a double bond with the (Z) isomerism. An increase was obtained in the antiproliferative activity of **44** (IC_{50} = 9.40 ± 0.64 μM, entry 9). On comparing structures **44** and (Z)-**43**, it is worth emphasizing that the introduction of the double bond in compound (Z)-**43** increased ≈ 4.5-fold the antiproliferative activity (IC_{50} = 9.40 ± 0.64 μM, entry 9 against IC_{50} = 42.0 ± 2.33 μM, entry 10).

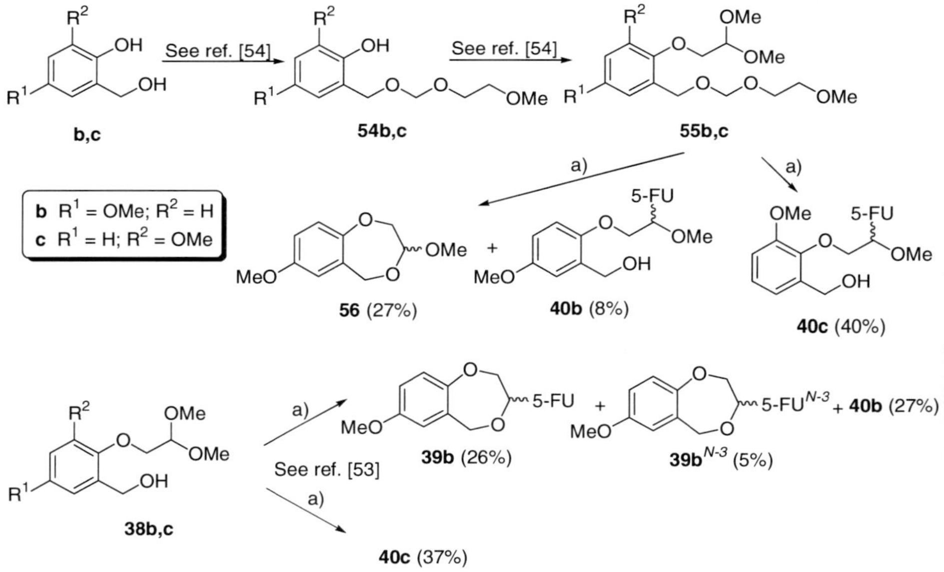

Scheme 14. Reagents: (a) 5-FU, HMDS, TCS, $SnCl_4/CH_2Cl_2$, MeCN. The identification tag **39b**$^{N\text{-}3}$ indicates that the 5-FU moiety is linked to the carbon chain through its *N*-3 atom.

Table 7. Antiproliferative activities, cell cycle dysregulation, and apoptosis induction in the MCF-7 human breast cancer cell line after treatment for 24 or 12, and 48 h for the compounds

Entry	Compound	IC$_{50}$ (μM)[a]	Cell Cycle (48 h)[b]			Apoptosis[c]	
			G$_0$/G$_1$	S	G$_2$/M	24 or 12 h	48 h
1	Control		68.39	12.04	19.57	1.07 $\pm$ 0.22	1.23 $\pm$ 0.13
2	40a[d]	18.5 $\pm$ 0.95	67.18	4.67	28.16	59.90 $\pm$ 2.65[e]	40.23 $\pm$ 1.98
3	40d[d]	18.0 $\pm$ 0.85	71.01	28.99	0.00	44.36 $\pm$ 2.01[e]	50.64 $\pm$ 2.24
4	40e[d]	16.0 $\pm$ 1.18	51.45	20.66	27.88	42.24 $\pm$ 1.89[e]	36.37 $\pm$ 1.68
5	41a	44.0 $\pm$ 1.26	64.51	25.39	10.10	3.60 $\pm$ 0.25[f]	2.06 $\pm$ 0.11
6	41d	18.0 $\pm$ 0.92	72.15	20.52	7.33	7.15 $\pm$ 0.97[f]	1.15 $\pm$ 0.12
7	41e	18.0 $\pm$ 1.05	72.45	18.17	9.38	2.71 $\pm$ 0.37[f]	1.86 $\pm$ 0.20
8	42	27.0 $\pm$ 1.13	63.71	29.67	6.62	3.17 $\pm$ 0.13[f]	1.68 $\pm$ 0.35
9	(*Z*)-43	9.40 $\pm$ 0.64	55.76	42.33	1.91	1.36 $\pm$ 0.25[f]	1.70 $\pm$ 0.15
10	44	42.0 $\pm$ 2.33	66.29	33.71	0.00	2.18 $\pm$ 0.27[f]	1.56 $\pm$ 0.53

[a]Data determined according to ref. [56].

[b]Data determined by flow cytometry [57].

[c]Apoptosis was determined using an annexin V-based assay [57]. The data indicate the percentage of cells undergoing apoptosis in each sample. All experiments were conducted in duplicate and gave similar results. The data are means $\pm$ SEM of three independent determinations.

[d]Data (antiproliferative activity, cell cycle distribution and apoptosis) taken from ref. [49].

[e]24 h.

[f]12 h.

Correlation (1) between antiproliferative activity of compounds **41a,d,c, 42** and (*Z*)-**43** and their calculated lipophilicities by the CDR option of the PALLAS 2.0 programme [58] (Table 8) was obtained:

$$p(\text{IC}_{50}) = 4.20\ (\pm 0.04) + 0.46\ (\pm 0.04)\ \text{clog } P$$

$$n = 5,\ r^2 = 0.976,\ s = 0.044,\ F_{1,3} = 124.26,\ \alpha < 0.001 \tag{1}$$

Outlier not included: **44**.

$p(\text{IC}_{50}) = -\log(\text{IC}_{50})$, bearing in mind that the higher the value of $p(\text{IC}_{50})$ the more potent is the compound, n is the number of compounds, r^2 is correlation coefficient, s is the standard deviation, F is the F ratio between the variances of observed and calculated activities, and data within parentheses are standard errors of estimate. In the derivation of equation (1) the more lipophilic compound **44** (Table 8, clog P = 1.84) was not included as it was found to be a misfit in the correlation. It could be hypothesized that the low antiproliferative of **44** is attributed to the high flexibility of its side-chain orientation.

Table 8. Antiproliferative activities in the MCF-7 human breast cancer cell line after treatment, and calculated lipophilicities for the compounds

	41a	41d	41e	42	(Z)-43	44
$p(IC_{50})^a$	4.36	4.74	4.74	4.57	5.03	4.38
clog P^b	0.32	1.06	1.26	0.87	1.76	1.84

[a] $p(IC_{50})$ = -log(IC_{50}), bearing in mind that the higher the value of $p(IC_{50})$ the more potent is the compound.

[b] Calculated by the CDR option of the PALLAS 2.0 programme [58].

It is well established that different anticancer drugs may exert their therapeutic effects by combining differentiating and cytotoxic actions in several types of cancer [59]. Genes that are altered in neoplasia affect three important biological routes that normally regulate the cell growing and the tissue homeostasis: cell cycle, apoptosis and differentiation. Although each of these routes can be defined by means of a unique set of molecular events, they are intimately interrelated in such a way that if one of them is disturbed profound consequences can be produced in the others [60]. The new compounds may therefore affect any of these routes in a more specific way, giving rise to the antitumour effect.

Once the antiproliferative activity was determined, it was decided to check the modifications that the different compounds provoked in the cell cycle. Such a study showed differences in the behaviour pattern depending on the structural changes carried out. While **40a** concentrated the cancerous cells in the G_2/M phase (Table 7, entry 2), **40d** gathered the cells in the S phase (Table 7, entry 3). Meanwhile, **8e** distributed the cancerous cells between the S and G_2/M phases (Table 7, entry 4). Nevertheless, compounds **41a**, **42**, **(Z)-43** and **44** concentrated the cells in the S phase, whilst **41d** and **41e** gathered them in the S and G_0/G_1 phases. When bromine or chlorine (compounds **41d** and **41e**, respectively) was introduced at position 5 of the benzene ring, the increase in the antitumour activity in relation to **41a** was accompanied by an increment of the percentage of cells that were accumulated in the G_0/G_1 phase of the cell cycle. There was also a significant diminution in the G_2/M phase in relation to the control cells. Compound **(Z)-43** was the most active (9.4 ± 0.64 µM) giving rise to an arrest of the cells in the S phase of the cell cycle. It promoted a diminution in the percentage of cells in the G_0/G_1 and the decrease up to total disappearance of cells in the G_2/M phase.

Later, apoptosis assays using an annexin V-based assay and flow cytometry at different times of treatment. In response to **40a**, **40d** and **40e** (Table 7, entries 2-

4), the percentage of apoptotic cells increased, from 1.07% in control cells to a maximum of 59.90% (**40a**), 44.36% (**40d**) and 42.24% (**40e**) apoptotic cells (24 h) at a concentration equal to their IC_{50} against the MCF-7 cell line. Nevertheless, compounds **41a**, **41d**, **41e**, **42**, (*Z*)-**43** and **44** gave rise to only very slight increments in the apoptotic cells as can be deduced from Table 7. Such augmentations were more evident in the first 12 h and for compounds **41a** and **41d**. The modifications were minimal after 48 h, **41d** being the structure where more apoptotic cells appeared (Table 7, entry 6). From the data shown in Table 7, it can be concluded that compounds **41a**, **41d**, **41e**, **42**, (*Z*)-**43** and **44** do not act preferentially through an apoptotic mechanism in human breast cancer cells.

Finally, our aim was to identify the compounds capable of inducing cell differentiation on human breast cancer cells MCF-7. Differentiated breast cancer cells display properties that are associated with lactation and include the generation of fat deposits within the cytoplasm [61]. The percentage of lipid positive cells was determined by Nile Red staining in a flow cytometer. Nile red is a specific fluorescent probe for quantifying the intracellular lipid contents by flow cytometry in mammalian cells [62].

All the compounds (except **41a**) caused an increase in lipid content over control levels after 3 days of treatment (Figure 2). Compound (*Z*)-**43** increased the percentage of lipids up to values of more than 6-fold than that of the untreated cells. Nevertheless, (*Z*)-**43** increased the percentage of cells in the S phase in a significant way, which might contradict the high level of differentiation. Although, G_1 arrest has been the centre of attention in differentiation, some reports are concerned with the involvement of G_2/M and S-phase arrest in this event [63]. Moreover, recent studies have demonstrated that purine nucleotides and nucleosides caused S-phase arrest and differentiation in human cells of chronic myelogenous leukaemia [64]. The duplication of the cellular genome during the S-phase of cell cycle is critical because during this process the cells are highly susceptible to the induction of differentiation [65].

Introduction of the bromine and chlorine atoms causes an increment of the differentiation levels from two to 4-fold in relation to the control. The arrest of cells in the G_0/G_1 phase by these compounds shows the passage to a non-proliferative quiescent state that implies the entrance into the differentiation process [66]. Others [67] have shown that novel quinolone compounds caused lipid droplet accumulation as a phenotypic marker of differentiation, loss of Ki67 antigen expression, a cell cycle marker indicative of the entrance into the G_0 phase, and reduced protein levels of the G_1 one.

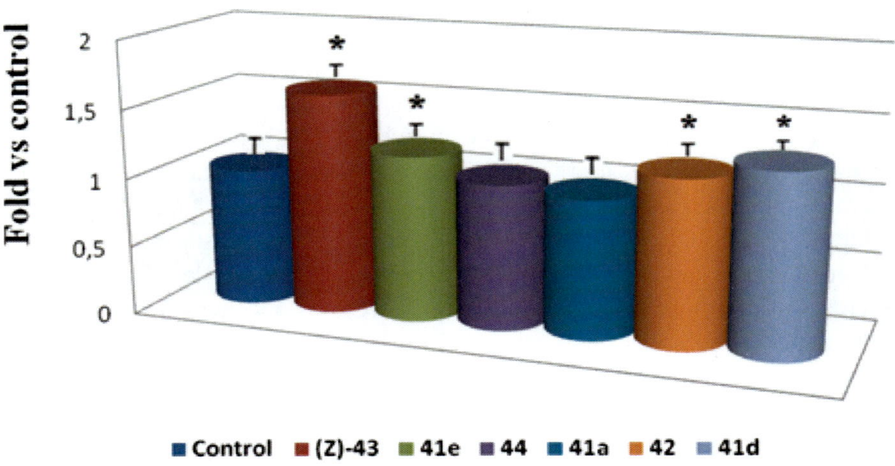

Figure 2. Quantification of the intracellular lipid contents Nile red staining by flow cytometry after treatment with the IC_{50} values of compound for 3 days. Percentage is expressed as the number of folds in comparison with non-treated MCF-7 cells. The histogram represents the mean of three determinations. All the data are significant at $P <$ 0.05 by Student's *t* test.

These data show that the mechanism by which such compounds exert their antiproliferative effect was the induction of differentiation in the MCF-7 human breast cancer cell line, instead of the induction of apoptosis or their cytotoxic action. Compounds led to the re-entry of the tumoural cells into the normal pathway of development and comprise a new category of experimental breast cancer differentiation agents [68].

CONCLUSION

In this review, we have presented the synthesis, mechanistic aspects and biological activity of various kinds of acyclic 5-FU *O,N*-acetals. The experimental findings provide evidence of specific antitumour activity of these new substances having the 5-FU moiety and warrant further evaluation in *in vivo* models of rahbomyosarcoma and breast cancer for future clinical applications. Finally, we hope that acyclic *O,N*-acetals bearing natural DNA bases will produce new types of antiviral and/or anticancer drugs.

ACKNOWLEDGMENTS

We thank the Instituto de Salud Carlos III [Fondo de Investigación Sanitaria (FIS) project no. PI10/00592] for financial support.

REFERENCES

[1]   Malet-Martino, M; Jolimaitre, P; Martino, R. The Prodrugs of 5-Fluorouracil. *Curr. Med. Chem.-Anti-Cancer Agents*, 2002, *2*, 267-310.

[2]   Schaeffer, HJ; Beauchamp, L; De Miranda, P; Elion, GB; Bauer, DJ; Collins, P. 9-(2-Hydroxyethoxymethyl)guanine activity against viruses of the herpes group, *Nature*, 1978, *272*, 583-585.

[3]   (a) Chu, CK; Suh, JJ; Mesbah, M; Cutler, SJ. Ring transformation reactions of C-nucleosides: facile synthesis of pyrazolo[1,5-a]pyrimidine and pyrazolo[1,5-a]triazine C-nucleosides. *Heterocyclic Chem.*, 1986, *23,* 349-352; (b) Chu, CK; Baker, DC. *Nucleosides and Nucleotides as Antitumor and Antiviral Agents*. Plenum Press: New York, 1993.

[4]   De Clercq, E; Sakuma, T; Baba, M; Pauwels, R; Balzarini, J; Rosenberg, I.; Holy, A. Antiviral activity of phosphonylmethoxyalkyl derivatives of purine and pyrimidines. *Antiviral Res.* 1987, *8*, 261-272.

[5]   Hitchcock, MJM; Jaffe, HS; Martin, JC; Stagg, RJ. Cidofovir, a new agent with potent antiherpes virus activity. *Antiviral Chem. Chemotherapy*, 1996, *7*, 115-127.

[6]   Kumar, R; Nath, M; Lorne, D. Tyrrell, J. Design and Synthesis of Novel 5-Substituted Acyclic Pyrimidine Nucleosides as Potent and Selective Inhibitors of Hepatitis B Virus. *J. Med. Chem.*, 2002, *45*, 2032-2040.

[7]   Balzarini, J; Pannecouque, C; Naesens, L; Andrei, G; Snoeck, R; De Clercq, E; Hockova, D; Holy, A. 6-[2-Phosphonomethoxy)Alkoxy]-2,4-Diaminopyrimidines: A New Class of Acyclic Pyrimidine Nucleoside Phosphonates with Antiviral Activity. *Nucleos. Nucleot. Nucl.*, 2004, *23*, 1321-1327.

[8]   Ajmera, S; Bapat, AR; Stephanian, E; Danenberg, PV. Synthesis and interaction with uridine phosphorylase of 5'-deoxy-4',5-difluorouridine, a new prodrug of 5-fluorouracil. *J. Med. Chem.*, 1988, *31*, 1094-1098.

[9]   Farquhar, D; Chen, R; Khan, S. 5'-[4-(Pivaloyloxy)-1,3,2-dioxaphosphorinan-2-yl]-2'-deoxy-5-fluorouridine: a membrane-permeating prodrug of 5-fluoro-2'-deoxyuridylic acid (FdUMP). *J. Med. Chem.*, 1995, *38*, 488-495.

[10] For a preliminary account of this work, see: (a) Gallo, MA; Espinosa, A; Campos, J; Entrena, A; Dominguez, JF; Camacho, E; Pineda, MJ; Gómez, JA. A Facile Synthetic Method for Pyrimidine Acyclonucleoside Analogues from Alkoxy-1,4-Diheterocycloheptanes. *Synlett*, 1993, *6*, 389-390; (b) Gallo, MA; Espinosa, A; Campos, J; Entrena, A; Pineda, MJ; Gómez, JA. Anticancer Pyrimidine Acyclonucleosides. *Il Farmaco,* 1995, *50*, 395-400. (c) Universidad de Granada, Eur. *Pat. Appl.* WO 91 17,147 (Cl. C07D239/54); *via Chem. Abstr.*, 1992, 117, 49156d.

[11] King, B. *Encyclopedia of Inorganic Chemistry.* John Wiley & Sons: New York, 1994.

[12] Choi, W-B; Wilson, LJ; Yeola, S; Liotta, DC; Schinazi, RF. *In situ* complexation directs the stereochemistry of *N*-glycosylation in the synthesis of thialanyl and dioxolanyl nucleoside analogs. *J. Am. Chem. Soc.*, 1991, *113*, 9377-9379.

[13] Wilson, LJ; Hager, MW; El-Kattan, YA; Liotta, DC. Nitrogen glycosylation reactions involving pyrimidine and purine nucleoside bases with furanoside sugars. *Synthesis*, 1995, 1465-1479.

[14] For the use of $BF_3 \cdot OEt_2$ as an effective catalyst for nucleoside formation, see Niedballa, U; Vorbrüggen, H. Synthesis of nucleosides. 11. General synthesis of *N*-glycosides. III. Simple synthesis of pyrimidine disaccharide nucleosides. *J. Org. Chem.*, 1974, *39*, 3664-3667.

[15] Vorbrüggen, H; Höfle, G. Nucleoside syntheses. XXIII. On the mechanism of nucleoside synthesis. *Chem. Ber.*, 1981, *114*, 1256-1268.

[16] (a) Smith, MB; March, J. March's Advanced Organic Chemistry. Reactions, Mechanisms, and Structure; 6th Edition. Wiley-Interscience: New York; 2007.

[17] Campos, J; Pineda, MJ; Gómez, JA; Entrena, A; Trujillo, MA; Gallo, MA; Espinosa, A. 5-Fluorouracil Derivatives. 1. Acyclonucleosides through a Tin(IV) Chloride-Mediated Regiospecific Ring Opening of Alkoxy-1,4-Diheteroepanes. *Tetrahedron*, 1996, *52*, 8907-8924.

[18] Espinosa, A; Entrena, A; Gallo, MA; Campos, J; Domínguez, JF; Camacho, E; Sánchez, I. Conformational Analysis of Some 1,4-Dioxepane Systems. 2. Methoxy-1,4-dioxepanes. *J. Org. Chem.*, 1990, *55,* 6018-6023.

[19] McCormick, JE; McElhinney, RS. Nucleoside analogs. Part 1. Some 5-fluorouracil *seco*-nucleosides and their hydrolysis by dilute acid. *J. Chem. Research (M)*, 1983, 176-177.

[20] Fluoropyrimidines are amongst the few options in the chemotherapeutic treatment of colorectal cancers.

[21] Braña, MF; Castellano, JM; Morán, M; Pérez de Vega, MJ; Romerdahl, CA; Quian, X-D; Bousquet, P; Ending, F; Schlick, E; Keilhauer, G. Bis-naphthalimides: a new class of antitumor agents. *Anticancer Drug Res.*, 1993, *8,* 257-268.

[22] Gómez, JA; Campos, J; Marchal, JA; Trujillo, MA; Melguizo, C; Prados, J; Gallo, MA; Aránega, A; Espinosa, A. Chemical Modifications on the Acyclic Moiety of 3-(2-Hydroxyethoxy)-1-Alkoxypropyl Nucleobases. 2. Differentiation and Growth Inhibition in Rhabdomyosarcoma Cells after Exposure to a Novel 5-Fluorouracil Acyclonucleoside. *Tetrahedron,* 1997, *53,* 7319-7334.

[23] For the regiospecific syntheses of 2-chloro-2'-deoxy-2'-fluoroadenosine (*N*-9-adenine derivative) and its *N*-7-isomer using trimethyl trifluoromethanesulfonate and tin(IV) chloride, respectively, see: Zaitseva, GV; Sivets, GG; Kazimierczuk, Z; Vilpo, JA; Mikhailopulo, IA. Convergent synthesis and cytostatic properties of 2-chloro-2'-deoxy-2'-fluoroadenosine and its *N*7-isomer. *Biorg. & Med. Chem. Lett.*, *1995, 5,* 2999-3002.

[24] Vorbrüggen, H.; Ruh-Pohlenz, C. Synthesis of Nucleosides. *Organic Reactions (New York)*, 2000, *55,* 1-630.

[25] Chenon, M-T; Pugmire, RJ; Grant, DM; Panzica, RP; Townsend, LB. Carbon-13 magnetic resonance. XXV. Basic set of parameters for the investigation of tautomerism in purines established from carbon-13 magnetic resonance studies using certain purines and pyrrolo[2,3-d]pyrimidines. *J. Am. Chem. Soc.*, 1975, *97,* 4627-4636.

[26] Espinosa, A; Gallo, MA; Campos, J; Gómez, JA. Diastereoselective Intramolecular Cyclization through the Triphenylphosphine/Carbon Tetrachloride System: Synthesis of Saturated 1,4-Dihetero Seven-Membered Cycloacetals. *Synlett*, 1995, *11,* 1119-1120.

[27] Hall, RH; Stern, ES. □□-Unsaturated aldehydes and related compounds. II. The reaction of □□-unsaturated aldehydes with unsaturated alcohols in the presence of alkali. *J. Chem. Soc.*, 1952, 4083-4085.

[28]   Taber, DF; Amedio, JC J.; Jung, K-Y. Phosphorus pentoxide/dimethyl sulfoxide/triethylamine (PDT): a convenient procedure for oxidation of alcohols to ketones and aldehydes. *J. Org. Chem.*, 1987, *52,* 5621-5622.

[29]   For the oxidation of a primary hydroxyl group of a carbohydrate to an acid carboxylic acid derivative (methyl gluconate) using DMSO and P_2O_5, see Onodera, K; Hirano, S; Kashimura, N. Oxidation of carbohydrates with dimethyl sulfoxide containing phosphorus pentaoxide. *J. Am. Chem. Soc.*, 1965, *87,* 4651-4652.

[30]   Corey, EJ; Suggs, JW. Pyridinium chlorochromate. Efficient reagent for oxidation of primary and secondary alcohols to carbonyl compounds. *Tetrahedron Lett.*, 1975, 2647-2650.

[31]   (a) Coates, WM; Corrigan, JR. Pyridine dichromate as an oxidizing agent. *Chem. Ind. (London)*, 1969, 1594; (b) Corey, EJ; Schmidt, G. Useful procedures for the oxidation of alcohols involving pyridinium dichromate in aprotic media. *Tetrahedron Lett.*, 1979, 399-402; (c) Czernecki, S; Georgoulis, C; Stevens, CL; Vijayaknmaran, K. Pyridinium dichromate oxidation. Modifications enhancing its synthetic utility. *Tetrahedron Lett.*, 1985, *26,* 1699-1702.

[32]   32. Lifshitz, E. Goidfarb, D; Vega, S; Luz, Z; Zimmermann, H. Deuterium and carbon-13 NMR of the solid polymorphism of benzenehexoyl hexa-n-hexanoate. *J. Am. Chem. Soc.*, 1987, *109,* 7280-7286.

[33]   (a) Bowden, IC; Heilbron, IM; Jones, ERH; Weedon, BCL. Acetylenic compounds. I. Preparation of acetylenic ketones by oxidation of acetylenic carbinols and glycols. *J. Chem. Soc.*, 1946, 39-45; (b) Bowers, A; Halsall, TG; Jones, ERH.; Lemin, AJ. Chemistry of the triterpenes and related compounds. XVIII. Elucidation of the structure of polyporenic acid C. *J. Chem. Soc.*, 1953, 2548-2560.

[34]   D'Amore ESG; Tollot, M; Stracca-Panca, V; Menegon, A; Mell, S; Ninfo, V. Therapy associated differentiation in rhabdomyosarcomas. *Modern Pathol.*, 1994, *7,* 69-75.

[35]   Crouch, GD; Kalebic, T; Tsokos, M; Hdman, L. Ara-C treatment leads to differentiation and reverses the transformed phenotype in a human rhabdomyosarcoma cell line. *J. Exp. Cell. Res.*, 1993, *204,* 210-216.

[36]   Melguizo, C; Prados, J; Fernández, JE; Vélez, C; Álvarez, L; Aránega, A. Actinomycin D causes multidrug resistance and differentiation in a human rhabdomyosarcoma cell line. *Cell. Mol. Biol.*, 1994, *40,* 137-145.

[37]   Shimada, H; Newton, WA; Soule, EH; Beltangady, MS; Maurerx, MS. Pathology of fatal rhabdomyosarcoma. Report from Intergroup Rhabdomyosarcoma Study (IRS-I and IRS-II). *Cancer*, 1987, *59,* 459-465.

[38] (a) Altmannsberger, M; Weber, K; Droste, R; Osborn, M. Desmin is a specific marker for rhabdomyosarcomas of human and rat origin. *Am. J. Pathol.*, 1985, *118*, 85-95; (b) Vélez, C; Muros, MA; Aránega AE; Fernández, JE; González, FJ; Álvarez, L; Aránega, A. Coexpression of intermediate filament proteins in the chick embryo heart. *Acta Anat.*, 1990, *139*, 226-233.

[39] Prados, J; Melguizo, C; Fernández, JE; Aránega, AE; Alvarez, L; Aránega, A. Actin, tropomyosin and □-actinin as markers of differentiation in human rhabdomyosarcoma cell lines induced with dimethyl sulfoxide. *Cell. Mol. Biol.*, 1993, *39*, 525-536.

[40] Pizzorno, G; Sun, Z; Handschumacher, RE. Aberrant cell cycle inhibition pattern in human colon carcinoma cell lines after exposure to 5-fluorouracil. *Biochem. Pharmacol.*, 1995, *49*, 553-557.

[41] Briefly, through FACScan we endeavour to monitor the cellular components by means of specific monoclonal antibodies for such components. This technique lies in the measurement of both the scattered laser light by cells and the emitted fluorescence by the cells labelled by a fluorescent antibody directed towards such a cellular component. Significance was determined by comparison of the means with Student's test. All differences were significant at $p < 0.001$.

[42] Aránega, A; Marchal, JA; Melguizo, C; Prados, J; Aránega, AE; Vélez, C; Fernández, JE; Arena, N; Álvarez, L. Low sample volume causes differentiation in human rhabdomyosarcoma cell line RD subjected to electroporation. *Cell. Mol. Biol.*, 1996, *42*, 1219-1227.

[43] (a) Lesuffleur, T; Kornowski, A; Luccioni, C; Muleris, M; Barbat, A; Beaumatin, J; Dussaulx, E; Dutrillaux, B; Zweibaum, A. Adaptation to 5-fluorouracil of the heterogeneous human colon tumor cell line HT-29 results in the selection of cells committed to differentiation. *Int. J. Cancer*, 1991, *49*, 721-730; (b) Lesuffleur, T; Kornowski, A; Augeron, C; Dussaulx, E; Barbat, A; Laboisse, C. Zweibum, *A*. Increased growth adaptability to 5-fluorouracil and methotrexate of HT-29 sub-populations selected for their commitment to differentiation. *Int. J. Cancer*, 1991, *49*, 731-737.

[44] (a) Lotan, R; Francis, GE; Freeman, CS; Waxman S. Differentiation therapy. *Cancer Res.*, 1990, *50*, 3453-3464; (b) Zupi, G; Marangolo, M; Arancia, G; Greco, C; Laudonio, N; Iosi, F; Formisano, G; Malorni, W. Modulation of the cytotoxic effect of 5-fluorouracil by N-methylformamide on a human colon carcinoma cell line. *Cancer Res.*, 1988, *48*, 6193-6200; (c) Waxman, S; Huang, Y; Scher, BM; Seller, M. Enhancement of differentiation and cytotoxicity of leukemia cells by combinations of

fluorinated pyrimidines and differentiation inducers: development of DNA double-strand breaks. *Biomed. Pharmacother.*, 1992, *46,* 183-192.

[45] (a) Richards, MA; Westcombe, AM; Love, SB; Littlejonhs, P; Ramirez, A.J. Influence of delay on survival in patients with breast cancer: a systematic review. *Lancet*, 1999, *353*, 1119-1126; (b) Norton, L. Adjuvant breast cancer therapy: current status and future strategies-growth kinetics and the improved drug therapy of breast cancer. *Semin. Oncol.*, 1999, *26*, 1–4; (c) Morrow, M; Jordan, VC; Takei, H; Gradishar, WJ; Pierce, LJ. Current controversies in breast cancer management. *Curr. Probl. Surg.*, 1999, *36*, 163–216; (d) Ruppert, JM; Wright, M; Rosenfeld, M; Grushcow, G; Bilbao, G. Curiel, DT; Strong, TV. Gene therapy strategies for carcinoma of the breast. *Breast Cancer Res. Treat.*, 1997, *44*, 93–114.

[46] Coultas, L; Strasser, A. The molecular control of DNA damage-induced cell death. *Apoptosis*, 2000, *5*, 491-507.

[47] Rasbridge, SA; Gillet, CE; Seymour, AM; Patel, K; Richards, MA; Rubens, RD; Millis, RR. The effects of chemotherapy on morphology, cellular proliferation, apoptosis and oncoprotein expression in primary breast carcinoma. *Brit. J. Cancer*, 1994, *70*, 335–341.

[48] Meier, C; De Clercq, E; Balzarini, J. Nucleotide delivery from cycloSaligenyl-3'-azido-3'-deoxythymidine monophosphates (cycloSal-AZTMP). *Eur. J. Org. Chem.*, 1998, 837–846.

[49] Saniger, E; Campos, JM; Entrena, A; Marchal, JA; Suárez, I; Aránega, A; Choquesillo, D; Niclós, J; Gallo, MA; Espinosa, A. Medium Benzene-fused Oxacycles with the 5-Fluorouracil Moiety: Synthesis, Antiproliferative Activities and Apoptosis Induction in Breast Cancer Cells. *Tetrahedron*, 2003, *59*, 5457–5467.

[50] 50. Ozaki, S; Watanabe, Y; Hoshiko, T; Nagase, T; Ogasawara, T; Furukawa, H; Uemura, A; Ishikawa, K; Mori, H; Hoshi, A; Iigo, M; Tokuzen, R. 5-Fluorouracil derivatives. X. Synthesis and antitumor activities of alpha-alkoxyalkyl-5-fluorouracils. *Chem. Pharm. Bull.*, 1986, *34*, 150-157.

[51] (a) Sampath, D; Plunkett, W. Design of new anticancer therapies targeting cell cycle checkpoint pathways. *Curr. Opin. Oncol.*, 2001, *13*, 484–490; (b) Gali-Muhtasib, H; Bakkar, N. Modulating cell cycle: current applications and prospects for future drug development. *Curr. Cancer Drugs Targets*, 2002, *2*, 309-336.

[52] (a) Saunders, DE; Lawrence, WD; Christensen, C; Wappler, NL; Ruan, H; Deppe, G. Paclitaxel-induced apoptosis in MCF-7 breast-cancer cells. *Int. J. Cancer*, 1997, *70*, 214–220; (b) Chadderton, A; Villeneuve, DJ; Gluck, S;

Kirwan-Rhude, AF; Gannon, BR; Blais, DE; Parissenti, AM. Role of specific apoptotic pathways in the restoration of paclitaxel-induced apoptosis by valspodar in doxorubicin-resistant MCF-7 breast cancer cells. *Breast Cancer Res. Tr.*, 2000, *59*, 231-244.

[53] Saniger, E; Campos, JM; Entrena, A; Marchal, JA; Boulaiz, H; Aránega, A; Gallo, MA; Espinosa, A. Neighbouring-group participation as the key step in the reactivity of acyclic and cyclic salicyl-derived *O,O*-acetals with 5-fluorouracil. Antiproliferative activity, cell cycle dysregulation and apoptotic induction of new *O,N*-acetals against breast cancer cells. *Tetrahedron*, 2003, *59*, 8017-8026.

[54] Saniger, E; Díaz-Gavilán, M; Delgado, B; Choquesillo, D; González-Pérez, JM; Aiello, S; Gallo, MA; Espinosa, A; Campos, JM. Substituent effects on the reaction mode between 2-hydroxybenzyl alcohol derivatives and MEM chloride: synthesis and mechanistic aspects of seven- and ten-membered benzo-fused *O,O*-acetals. *Tetrahedron*, 2004, *60*, 11453-11464.

[55] Hager, MW; Liotta, DC. Cyclization protocols for controlling the glycosidic stereochemistry of nucleosides. Application to the synthesis of the antiviral agent 3'-azido-3'-deoxythymidine (AZT). *J. Am. Chem. Soc.*, 1991, *113*, 5117-5119.

[56] Cellai, C; Laranzana, A; Vannucchi, AM; Caporale, R; Paglierani, M; Di Lollo, S; Pancrazzi, A; Paoletti, F. Growth inhibition and differentiation of human breast cancer cells by the PAFR antagonist WEB-2086. *Br. J. Cancer*, 2006, *94*, 1637-1642.

[57] Wang, JL; Liu, D; Zhang, ZJ; Shan, S; Han, X; Srinivasula, SM; Croce, CM; Alnemri, ES; Huang, Z. Structure-based discovery of an organic compound that binds Bcl-2 protein and induces apoptosis of tumor cells. *Proc. Natl. Acad. Sci. USA*, 2000, *97*, 7124-7129.

[58] Pallas Frame Module, a prediction tool of physicochemical parameters, is supplied by CompuDrug Chemistry Ltd, PO Box 23196, Rochester, NY 14696, USA.

[59] (a) Marchal, JA; Prados, J; Melguizo, C; Fernández, JE; Vélez, C; Álvarez, L; Aránega, A. Actinomycin D treatment leads to differentiation and inhibits proliferation in rhabdomyosarcoma cells. *J. Lab. Clin. Med.*, 1997, *130*, 42-50; (b) Camarasa, MV; Castro-Galache, MD; Carrasco-García, E; García-Morales, P; Saceda, M; Ferragut, J. Differentiation and drug resistance relationships in leukemia cells. *J. Cell. Biochem.*, 2005, *94*, 98-108.

[60] Corn, PG; El-Deiry, WS. Derangement of growth and differentiation control in oncogenesis. *BioEssays*, 2002, *24*, 83-90.

[61]   Seewaldt, VL; Kim, JH; Parker, MB; Dietze, FC; Srinivasan, KV; Caldwell, LF. Dysregulated Expression of Cyclin D1 in Normal Human Mammary Epithelial Cells Inhibits All-*trans*-Retinoic Acid-Mediated G0/G1-Phase Arrest and Differentiation *in Vitro*. *Exp. Cell Res.*, 1999, *249*, 70-85.

[62]   Greenspan, P; Mayer, EP; Fowler, SD. Nile red: a selective fluorescent stain for intracellular lipid droplets. *J. Cell Biol.*, 1985, *100*, 965-973.

[63]   (a) Rapaport, E. Treatment of human tumor cells with ADP or ATP yields arrest of growth in the S phase of the cell cycle. *J. Cell. Physiol.*, 1983, *114*, 279-283; (b) Gorin, NC; Estey, E; Jones, RJ; Levitsky, HI; Borrello, I; Slavin, S. New Developments in the Therapy of Acute Myelocytic Leukemia. *Hematology*, 2000, 69-89.

[64]   Moosavi, MA; Yazdanparast, R; Lotfi, A. GTP induces S-phase cell-cycle arrest and inhibits DNA synthesis in K562 cells but not in normal human peripheral lymphocytes. *J. Biochem. Mol. Biol.*, 2006, *39*, 492-501.

[65]   Huang, M; Wang, Y; Collins, M; Mitchell, BS; Graves, LM. A771726 induces differentiation of human myeloid leukemia K562 cells by depletion of intracellular CTP pools. *Mol. Pharmacol.*, 2002, *62*, 463-472.

[66]   Marchal, JA; Prados, J; Melguizo, C; Gómez, JA; Campos, J; Gallo, MA; Espinosa, A; Arena, N; Aránega, A. GR-891: a novel 5-fluorouracil acyclonucleoside prodrug for differentiation therapy in rhabdomyosarcoma cells. *Br. J. Cancer*, 1999, *79*, 807-813.

[67]   Martirosyan, AR; Rahim-Bata, R; Freeman, AB; Clarke, CD; Howard, RL; Strobl, JS. Differentiation-inducing quinolines as experimental breast cancer agents in the MCF-7 human breast cancer cell model. *Biochem. Pharmacol.*, 2004, *68*, 1729-1738.

[68]   Díaz-Gavilán, M; Conejo-García, A; Cruz-López, O; Núñez, MC; Choquesillo-Lazarte, D; González-Pérez, JM; Rodríguez-Serrano, F; Marchal, JA; Aránega, A; Gallo, MA; Espinosa, A; Campos, JM. Synthesis and Anticancer Activity of (*RS*)-9-(2,3-Dihydro-1,4-Benzoxathiin-3-ylmethyl)-9*H*-Purines. *ChemMedChem*, 2008, *3*, 127-135.

In: Fluorouracil
Editors: A. Longinho and S. Dobreiro

ISBN: 978-1-62081-970-8
© 2012 Nova Science Publishers, Inc.

Chapter II

5-FLUOROURACIL AND ITS DERIVATIVES: SYNTHESIS, HEALTH EFFECTS AND CHEMOTHERAPY

Saurabh Garg[1], Nancy Gupta[1], Neeraj Shakya[1], Babita Agrawal[2] and Rakesh Kumar[*,1]

[1]Department of Laboratory Medicine and Pathology, Faculty of Medicine and Dentistry, University of Alberta, Edmonton, AB, Canada
[2]Department of Surgery, Faculty of Medicine and Dentistry, University of Alberta, Edmonton, AB, Canada

ABSTRACT

5-FU (5-fluorouracil, sold as Adrucil), a pyrimidine analog, has been widely used in the treatment of various cancers, including breast cancer, colorectal cancer, and cancers of digestive tract. Despite serious toxicity and considerable side effects, such as cardiotoxicity, ocular toxicity, hepatotoxicity and haematological toxicity, it is one of the first cancer treatments due to lack of better treatment options. Analogs of 5-FU have been studied as antimycotic, antimalarial, antineoplastic, antibacterial and antiviral (anti-HIV and anti- HBV) and anticancer agents. Newer analogs of 5-FU may prove effective and safe alternate of 5-FU for cancer treatment, in addition to their use in other diseases/disorders.

Introduction

INTRODUCTION

5-Fluorouracil (5-FU), a pyrimidine analog, is widely used as an antineoplastic agent against various types of cancers such as colorectal, breast, pancreatic, hepatoma, gastrointestinal, head and neck cancer.[1] 5-FU acts primarily as thymidylate synthase (TS) inhibitor, which blocks synthesis of thymidine, a pyrimidine nucleoside essential for DNA replication.[2] Nucleoside derivatives of 5-fluorouracil have also proven as potent anticancer agents. 5-Fluoro-2'-deoxyuridine (FUDR), an antineoplastic antimetabolite agent, is used for the treatment of colon cancer.[3] Other 5-FU derivatives such as Ftorafur and Doxifluridine have potential for renal, gastric, colorectal, breast and prostate cancers. [4] 5-FU and related derivatives proved to be a boon for various cancer patients, however, these TS inhibitory anticancer agents also have toxic effects on healthy tissue. The adverse effects include mild reversible myopathy, neuropathy, myelotoxicity, thrombocytopenia, neutropenia, mucositis, diarrhea, damage to bone marrow cells, blood cells, the intestinal lining, and multi-organ failure leading to death.[5] Apart from the serious side effects, resistance to 5-FU has been reported in cancer cells which poses significant limitations in the clinical use of 5-FU and also alarms for possible resistance to other nucleoside agents.[6] In light of increasing number of cancer patients and to overcome the hurdles of toxicity and resistance, there is an urgent need to find novel and effective chemotherapeutic strategy to combat various cancers.

5-FU analogs have also demonstrated significant antiviral and antibacterial activities. For example, 5-fluoro-3'-thiacytidine (FTC) is an effective compound in the treatment of human-immunodeficiency virus (HIV) and hepatitis B virus (HBV) infections. [7] This chapter aims to describe synthesis, chemotherapeutic and biological properties of 5-FU and its various derivatives.

5-FLUOROURACIL (ADRUCIL, EFUDEX, FLOUROPLEX)

5-FU was rationally designed and synthesized in 1957 by Heidelberger and co-workers on the basis of the observation that rat hepatomas use radiolabeled uracil more avidly than nonmalignant tissue.[8,9] It was a finding that suggested difference in enzymatic pathways used for uracil metabolism in normal vs. malignant cells. In this antimetabolite, an isosteric fluorine atom replaces the hydrogen atom at the C-5 position of uracil.[10] This molecule was designed to occupy the active sites of enzyme targets, thereby blocking metabolism in malignant cells. Even though 5-FU was first discovered over four decades ago, it remained a key anticancer drug as of today to treat various types of malignancies.[11] 5-FU is toxic, however, its efficacy, broad antitumor activity and synergism with other anticancer drugs makes it one of the most widely used agents against tumors including carcinomas of breast, gastrointestinal tract, renal, head and neck.[12,13]

5-FU gets converted to its active metabolites and demonstrates antitumor activity by three main mechanisms: a) 5-fluorouridine triphosphate (FUTP) that gets incorporated into cellular RNA instead of uridine triphosphate (UTP),[14,15] b) 5-fluorodeoxyuridine triphosphate (FdUTP), which is incorporated into DNA instead of deoxythymidine triphosphate (dTTP),[16,17] and c) 5-fluoro-2'-deoxyuridine-5'-monophosphate (5-FdUMP) inhibits the activity of thymidylate synthase (TS) in the ternary complex.[18] Among these mechanisms, TS is the main target for the action of 5-FU since thymidine is the only nucleotide precursor specific to DNA. In tumor cells TS and 2'-deoxyuridine-5'-monophosphate (dUMP) form a ternary complex, which transfers a methyl group from 5,10-methylene tetrahydrofolate ($C_{H2}THF$) on carbon 5 of dUMP and forms thymidine-5'-monophosphate (dTMP). Upon exposure with 5-FU and formation of adequate 5-FdUMP, the methyl transfer does not take place because the fluorine atom in the C5 position of 5-FdUMP is much more tightly bound than hydrogen. The enzyme is then trapped in a slowly reversible ternary complex and formation of dTMP is blocked. This leads to decrease in the availability of thymidine-5'-triphosphate (dTTP) for DNA replication and repair. TS inhibition leads to inhibition in cellular proliferation and also activates programmed cell death pathways.[19]

5-FU is used in many dosage regimens alone or as adjuvant therapy. It is given via intravenously (i.v.) push or bolus, or as continuous infusion principally for the treatment of colorectal cancers and pancreatic endocrine tumors.[20] It is also recommended topically as a cream for treating actinic keratoses and certain skin basal cell carcinomas. Generally, 12 mg/kg doses are administered i.v. once daily for 4 successive days. If no toxicity is observed, 6 mg/kg is given on the 6th, 8th, 10th and 12th days unless toxicity occurs. [21] Maximum recommended dose of 5-FU is 800 mg/day.

5-FU is metabolized primarily in liver via two routes: a) the anabolic route which gives rise to active metabolites; only 1-3% of the original dose of 5-FU mediates the cytotoxic effects through anabolic action, b) the catabolic route, which inactivates 5-FU and leads to its elimination from the organism[19]; 80-85% of 5-FU is catabolized to inactive metabolites by dihydropyrimidine dehydrogenase (DPD).[22] 5-FU has a short plasma half-life (10–20 min) *in vivo* and possess low bioavailability .[23]

5-FU exhibits serious toxicity and side effects. The degree and severity depends on the amount and schedule of the administration. The adverse effects of 5-FU include haematological toxicity (myelosuppression, leukocytopenia, anemia, thrombocytopenia, neutropenia, severe alopecia, dermatitis, atrophy and pigmentation of skin), immunosuppression, hand-foot syndrome, cardiotoxicity, ocular toxicity and hepatotoxicity. [24-26]

SYNTHESIS OF 5-FU

Two main routes have been reported for the synthesis of 5-FU in the literature (scheme 1). [27]

1. *Fluorination of uracil with CF₃OF*. This method includes reaction of uracil (**1**) with a mixture of trifluoroacetic acid (TFA) and water and a solution of CF_3OF in $CFCl_3$ at -78 °C in a pressure bottle. This procedure affords 5-FU (**2**) in 85% yield.
2. *Fluorination of uracil with fluorine*. In this method fluorine gas diluted liberally with nitrogen is passed into a vigorously stirred solution of uracil (**1**) in water at room temperature to yield 5-FU in 55% yield.

Reagents and conditions: (i) TFA/H_2O, CF_3OF/$CFCl_3$, -78 ° C (ii) F_2-N_2/ H_2O, r.t.

Several structural modifications in 5-FU have been investigated to reduce its toxic effects, and enhance pharmacological and pharmacokinetic properties. Some promising derivatives of 5-FU and their discovered biological properties are described as follows.

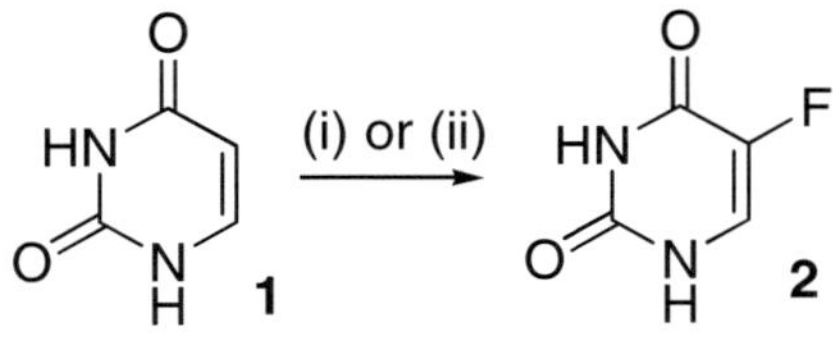

Scheme 1.

FLUCYTOSINE (5-FC)

5-FC or 5-fluorocytosine (**4**), a cytosine analogue of 5-FU, was investigated in 1957 [28] as a potential antitumour agent but was found to be not sufficiently active against tumours. [29] It can be used in combination with other anticancer agents for colorectal carcinoma. [30,31]

In 1968, however, it proved to be a potent antimycotic compound. [32,33] 5-FC itself has no antifungal activity, but after it has been taken up by susceptible fungal cells, it is converted in to 5-FU by the enzyme cytosine permease.[34] 5-FU is further converted to metabolites FUMP and FdUMP, which inhibit fungal RNA and DNA synthesis, respectively. [35] Monotherapy with 5-FC is limited because of the frequent development of resistance. [36] 5-FC in combination with other antifungal drugs, is used to treat severe systemic mycoses, such as cryptococcosis, candidosis, chromoblastomycosis, aspergillosis.

The recommended daily oral dose of 5FC is 50-150 mg/kg/day.[37] 5-FC is absorbed easily and rapidly. Its bioavailability is almost 90%. Peak serum concentration is achieved in 1-2 h. It is mainly excreted by the kidneys. [38] The half-life of FC in patients with normal renal function is 4-5 h. [37] Side effects associated with FC include hepatotoxicity, bone-marrow depression and gastrointestinal problems such as nausea, diarrhea, vomiting and diffused abdominal pain.[39,40] Like 5-FU, these side effects are concentration dependent, predictable and avoidable with close monitoring to maintain 5-FC concentration <100 mg/L.[41]

SYNTHESIS OF FLUCYTOSINE

5-FC synthesis is outlined in scheme 2. A reaction of trifluoromethylhypofluorite in trichlorofluoromethane with cytosine in methanol at -78 °C afforded 5-FC in 85% yield.42]

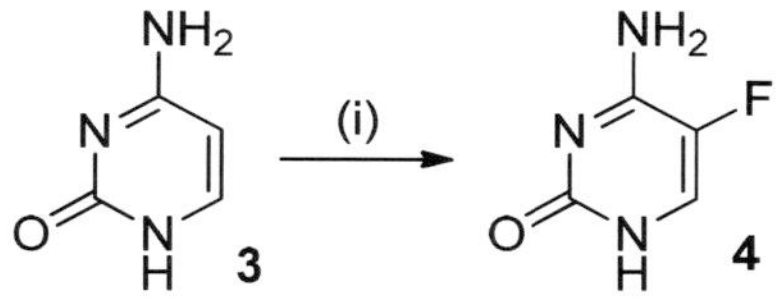

Scheme 2.

Reagent and conditions: (i) $CF_3OF/CFCl_3$, MeOH, -78 °C, 5 min.

5-FLUORO OROTIC ACID (5-FOA)

5-FOA (**11**) is a 6-carboxy analog of 5-FU. It has potent antimalarial activity both *in vitro* (IC_{50} = 6 nM) and *in vivo* against chloroquine-susceptible as well as chloroquine-resistant strains of *Plasmodium falciparum*.[43,44] 5-FOA is converted into 5-FU by OMP decarboxylase and leads eventually to the accumulation of a toxic metabolite 5-fluoro-2' deoxyuridylate, which inactivates thymidylate synthase in *P. falciparum* and also gets incorporated into nucleic acid.[45,46] 5-FOA inhibits proliferation of the mammalian cells and is no longer used as an antimalarial agent due to toxicity issues. [43]

SYNTHESIS

5-Fluoroorotic acid can be synthesized in 90% yield (scheme-3) by acidic treatment of ethyl-2-mercapto-4-hydroxy-5-fluoro-6-pyrimidine carboxylate (**10**). Compound **10** was obtained by the coupling reaction of S-ethylthiouronium bromide (**6**) with potassium diethylfluorooxaloacetate (**9**). The precursor material **6** was prepared starting from $BaCO_3$ via thiourea 3. The synthesis of **9** was conducted using ethyl oxalate as a starting material (scheme-3).[47]

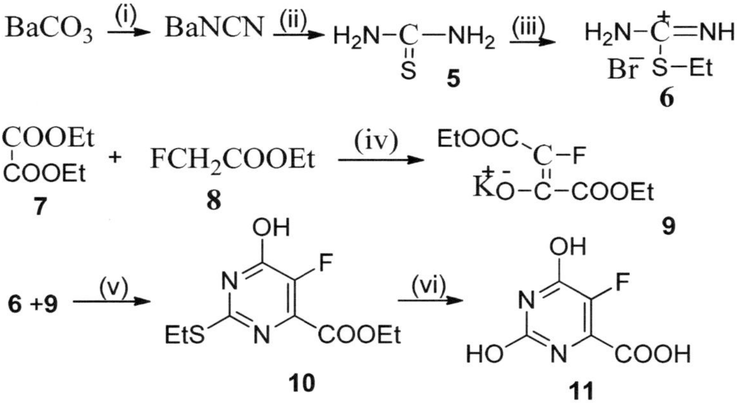

Scheme 3.

Reagent and conditions: (i) NH_3 (ii) H_2S/CO_2 (iii) EtOH, reflux, 12 h (iv) KOEt , r. t. (v) a) K, abs. EtOH, reflux, 2 h b) HCl (vi) conc. HCl, reflux, 4 h.

In order to reduce side effects and prolong half-life, some lipophilic groups were attached at different positions of FU and some of the novel derivatives of 5-FU possessing broader spectrum of antitumor activity with increased lipophilicity and fewer toxic side effects have been reported.

N-1 SUBSTITUTED 5-FU DERIVATIVES

Carmofur

Carmofur (1-hexylcarbamoyl-5-fluorouracil, HCFU) (**12**) was developed in the 1970s as an antineoplastic agent.[48] Compared to 5-FU, it has potent antitumor activity *in vitro*, and is less toxic clinically [49,50]. Carmofur has also been used as adjuvant chemotherapy for colorectal and breast cancer. [51] After oral administration, carmofur converts to 5-FU either enzymatically or non-enzymatically in the human body exerting its antitumor effect. Leukoencephalopathy has been reported as a serious side effect with its use.[52]

Synthesis

As depicted in scheme-4, carmofur can be synthesized in 95% yield by the treatment of 5-FU (2) with hexyl isocyanate in pyridine at 90°C. [53]

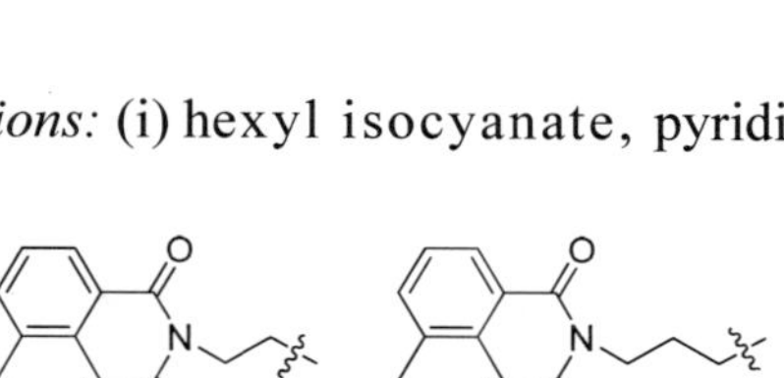

Scheme 4.

Reagent and conditions: (i) hexyl isocyanate, pyridine, 90°C, 1 h.

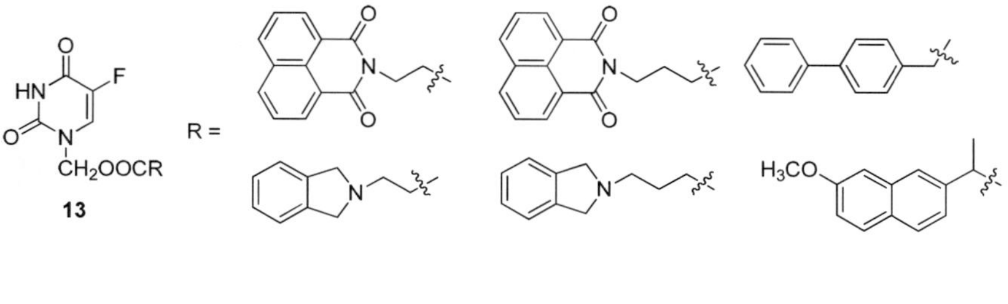

N-1-ESTERS OF 5-FU

N-1 ester modifications did not proved to be very potent as antitumor agents. Among various compounds investigated, **13** exhibited IC_{50} in the range of 3.7 to >50 μM (Chart 1). [5]

N-3 SUBSTITUTED 5-FU DERIVATIVES

N-3-O-toluyl-fluorouracil (tofluding, TFU, **14**), a prodrug of 5-FU, was developed by Kametani in 1980s, as a lipophilic potential anti-tumor drug. [54] Tofluding was effective against various tumors with fewer side effects both *in vitro* and *in vivo*.[55] In the body, it is selectively metabolized to 5-FU in the tumor cells by cytosolic enzymes. Tofluding possesses longer plasma half-life as compared to 5-FU. [56]

Synthesis

Tofluding (**14**) was synthesized by acylation of 5-FU (2) with 2-methylbenzoyl chloride in pyridine at room temperature (scheme 5). [57]

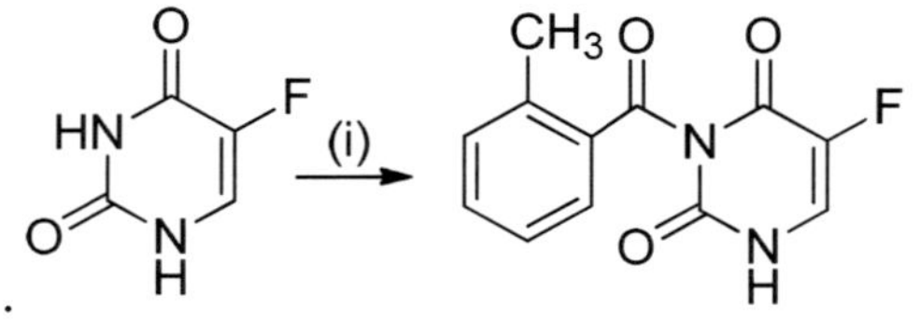

Scheme 5.

Reagent and conditions: (i) 2-Methylbenzoyl chloride, dry pyridine, r.t.

N-1,N-3 DISUBSTITUTED 5-FU DERIVATIVES

1,3-Bis(tetrahydro-2-furanyl) derivative of 5-FU (Thf$_2$-FU,**18**) was reported to inhibit various murine carcinomas in the range of 27 to 50% inhibition at 0.15

mmol/Kg dose. Thf$_2$-FU possesses similar activity to that of ftorafur (described below) against murine solid tumors but had lower toxicity.

Synthesis

The target compound **18** was synthesized in 81% yield by reacting Thf-OAc (**16**) with silylated 5-FU (**15**) under N$_2$ atmosphere. 3-Thf-FU (**17**) was also formed as side product in this reaction (Scheme 6).[58]

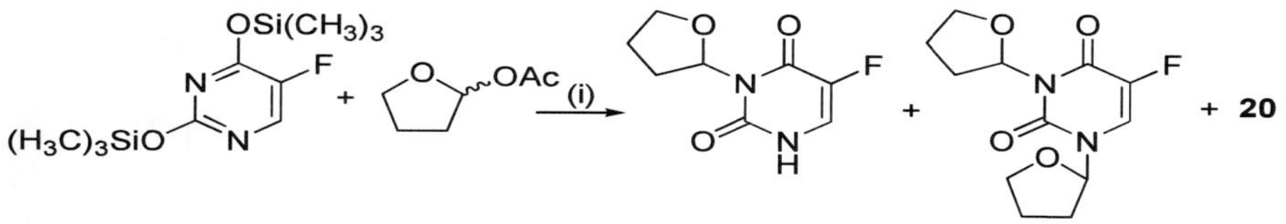

Scheme 6.

Reagent and conditions: (i) SnCl4, CH$_2$Cl$_2$, r.t., 3 h.

3-Thf-FU (**17**) was evaluated against AH-130 carcinoma in rats where it showed 45% and 80% inhibition at dose of 0.15 mmol/Kg and 0.45 mmol/Kg, respectively, but at higher dose it showed toxicity to normal body growth of rats.[58]

FTORAFUR

Ftorafur or tegafur (**20**) is a N-1-tetrahydrofuranyl analog of 5-FU. It was first developed in Japan as an oral anticancer agent. It is clinically used for lung, gastric, colorectal, and breast cancers. Ftorafur is a prodrug and is slowly metabolized to FU, which after conversion into active metabolites inhibits thymidylate synthase and RNA, DNA synthesis as described previously. Its oral dose is 400 mg/day. [59]

After intravenous administration, tegafur is converted into 5-FU spontaneously by cytochrome p-450 enzyme (CYP2A6 in human) or by thymidine phosphorylase present in liver, small intestine and tumor tissues. Oral administration of tegafur does not show sufficient antitumor effects because of relatively lower 5-FU concentrations. The intravenous single bolus injection of tegafur causes severe diarrhea, mucositis and central neurotoxicity. Gastrointestinal toxicities rarely occur with tegafur. [60]

Synthesis of Ftorafur

Ftorafur was obtained in 67% yield when 5-FU (**2**) was heated with 2-t-butoxytetrahydrofuran (**19**) in DMF at 150-155 °C for 5 hours. In this reaction, 5-fluoro-1,3-bis(2-tetrahydrofuryl)-uracil (**18**) is also obtained as a minor product that can be easily converted quantitatively into ftorafur in presence of acetic acid (scheme-7).[61]

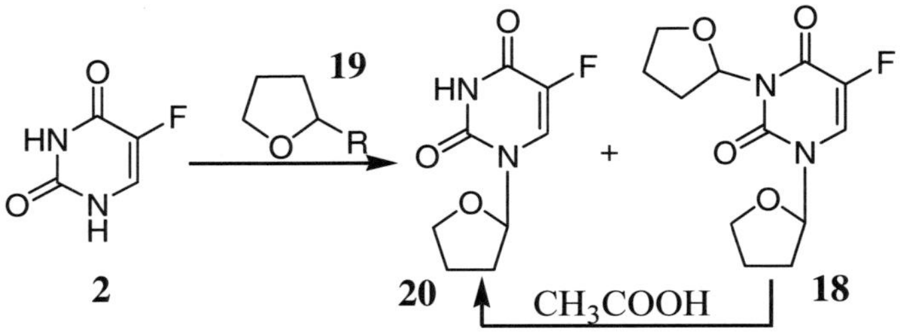

Scheme 7.

Reagent and conditions: (i) DMF, 150-155 ° C, 5 h.

NUCLEOSIDES ANALOGUES OF 5-FU

5-FU undergoes quick degradation and inactivation by dihydropyrimidine dehydrogenase (DPD) *in vivo*. To address this major limitation and improve the effectiveness, various nucleoside derivatives of 5FU have been developed. [62]

FLOXURIDINE (FUDR)

FUDR or 5-fluoro-2'-deoxyuridine (**22**) is a pyrimidine nucleoside analog of 5-FU. According to an *in vitro* study, FUDR is at least 100-fold more active than 5-FU at equimolar concentrations when examined in a panel of human cancer cell lines [62] FUDR was approved by FDA in 1970 for the treatment of hepatic colon metastases, breast and colorectal cancer.[63]

Floxuridine is metabolized to 5-FU in liver and then to 5-fluorodeoxyuridine monophosphate (F-dUMP) and fluorouridine triphosphate (FUTP). 5-FU inhibits uracil riboside phophorylase, which prevents the utilization of uracil in RNA synthesis. The monophosphate (F-dUMP) inhibits the enzyme thymidylate synthetase, which leads to the inhibition of methylation of deoxyuridylic acid to thymidylic acid, thus interfering in DNA synthesis. [64] FUDR is water-soluble and is easily transported across plasma membrane. When administered by slow, continuous, intra-arterial infusion, it is converted to monophosphate form. [62. The major side effects of FUDR include fatigue, diarrhea, nausea, and vomiting. [62]

Synthesis

The synthesis of FUDR (**22**) has been reported in 86% yield by the fluorination of the blocked 2'-deoxyuridine (**21**) using fluorinating agents such as CF_3OF in $CFCl_3$ or molecular fluorine as outlined in scheme 8. [65]

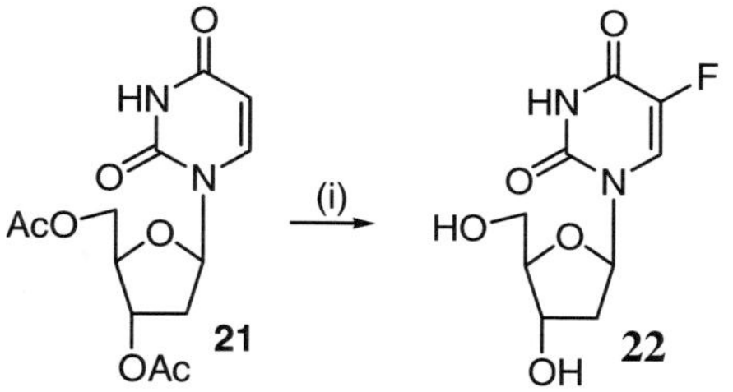

Scheme 8

Reagent and conditions: (i) CF_3OF in $CFCl_3$ in $CHCl_3$ -78 $^\circ$ C, 1 h or F_2.

BETA-D-5FDC

Beta-D-5FDC or 5-fluoro-2-deoxycytidine (**28**) is a DNA methylation inhibitor, which is rapidly and sequentially converted to 5-fluoro-2'-deoxyuridine, 5-fluorouracil, and 5-fluorouridine.[66,67] It is still being evaluated as a DNA methyltransferase inhibitor clinically. [68,69a] It is used as a prodrug and is converted by intracellular deaminases to FUDR and then to 5-fluorouracil, and 5-fluorouridine. [69b] FDC leads to potential toxic products and has lesser value as a drug.

Synthesis

Beta-D-5FDC (**28**) has been synthesized by the coupling reaction of 5-fluorocytosine (**4**) with 2-deoxy-3,5-di-O-p-toluoyl-D-ribofuranosyl chloride (**25**) as described in scheme 9. Compound **4** is refluxed with a 10% excess of p-toluoyl chloride to obtain **23** Conversion of **23** to N-4-p-toluoyl-5-fluorocytosine mercury **24** was carried out by treating it with mercuric acetate in ethanol in 94% yield. Condensation of **24** with 2-deoxy-3,5-di-O-p-toluoyl-D-ribofuranosyl chloride (**25**) in hot toluene yielded an anomeric mixture of nucleosides **26** (40%) and **27** (15%). Treatment of the obtained anomers with hot alcoholic ammonia or hot sodium methoxide in methanol afforded target compound **28** in 89% yield. [70]

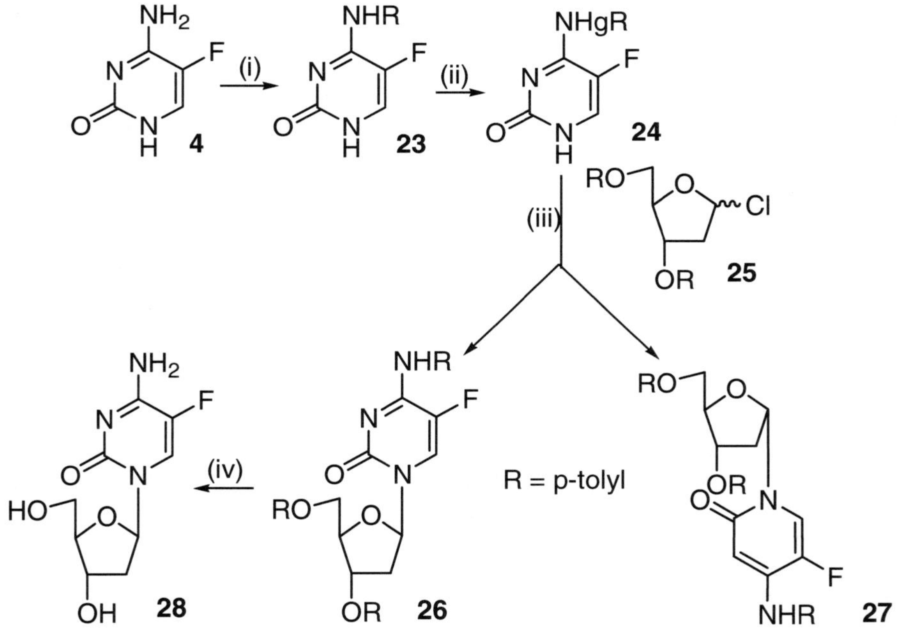

Scheme 9.

Reagent and conditions: (i) p-tolyl-chloride, pyridine, reflux, 5 h. (ii) mercuric acetate, ethanol, DMF, 100 ° C (iii) a) 3,5-di-(O-p-toluoyl)-2-deoxy-D-ribofuranosyl chloride, toluene, r.t., 45 min. b) 30% aqueous KI, 12 h (iv) 15% NH3, ethanol. r. t. 16h.

DOXIFLURIDINE

Doxifluridine or 5'-deoxy-5-fluorouridine (*33*) was synthesized by Cook et al in 1979. [71] It is an oral prodrug of the 5-FU [72]. Doxifluridine was designed to prevent the rapid degradation of 5-FU by dihydropyrimidine dehydrogenase in the gut wall. It is converted into 5-FU in the presence of pyrimidine nucleoside phosphorylase in the tumors [73]. Doxifluridine is used in breast, colorectal and gastric cancers.[73-75]

Doxifluridine is an oral prodrug that is metabolized to 5-FU by thymidine phosphorylase. 5-FU then acts by the mechanisms as described in the 5-FU section. It is less toxic than systemically administered 5-FU, as the conversion of doxifluridine into 5-FU takes place mainly in the tumor tissue.[74]

Doxifluridine is administered orally in the form of tablet or solution at a dose of 600-1000 mg three times daily. Doxifluridine is rapidly absorbed with a lag time of less than 20 min. The mean elimination half-life ($t_{1/2}$) is 32-45 min in the dose range of 600-1000 mg three times per day. [76]

The side effects of doxifluridine include diarrhea, mucositis, peripheral neurotoxicity, cardiac toxicity, nausea and vomiting. [75,77]

Synthesis

Synthesis of Doxifluridine has been achieved from 5-fluorouridine (**29**). 5-Fluorouridine (**29**) was first converted into a isopropylidene derivative **30** which upon treatment with methyltriphenoxyphosphonium iodide in DMF gave 5'-iodo compound **31**. Reduction of the 5'-iodo substituent of **31** was carried out using palladium on carbon as catalyst for 1.5 h to yield **32**. The obtained nucleoside **32** was deprotected using 90% trifluoroacetic acid to afford doxifluridine (**33**) in overall 56% yield from **29** (scheme-10). [71]

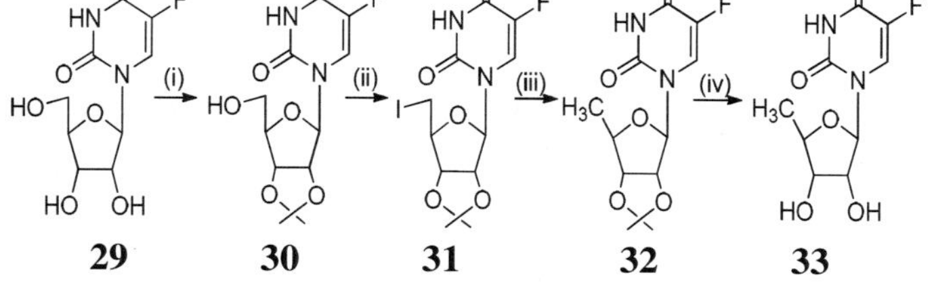

Scheme 10.

Reagent and conditions: (i) Propanone, HCl, MeOH, reflux, 1 h (ii) methyltriphenoxyphosphonium iodide, DMF, r. t., 50 min. (iii) 5% H_2-Pd/C, triethylamine, methanol, atm. pressure, 1.5 h (iv) 90% aqueous TFA, r.t., 1 h.

CAPECITABINE

Capecitabine or N-4-pentyloxycarbonyl-5'-deoxy-5-fluorocytidine (**37**) was approved by the US Food and Drug Administration in 2005. It is converted to 5-FU in tumor cells by thymidine phosphorylase. In contrast to 5-FU, capecitabine induced cardiotoxicity, including angina and myocardial infarction has not been reported frequently.[69]

Capecitabine has been widely used for gastric, colorectal, breast, head and neck cancers all over the world except in Japan, where it has not been approved.[69,74]

Orally administered capecitabine is first converted to 5'-deoxy-5-fluorocytidine by carboxylesterase and then to FUDR by cytidine deaminase in the liver and tumor tissues. Finally FUDR is converted to 5-FU by dThd phosphorylase in tumor cells. [4]

The National Comprehensive Cancer Network guidelines recommend 1000–1250 mg dose of capecitabine twice daily when it is given as monotherapy. In the case of rectal cancer, the recommended dose of capecitabine is 850 mg twice daily. Capecitabine is absorbed by the gastrointestinal tract followed by its conversion to 5-FU in three sequential enzymatic reactions, as stated above. The bioavailability of capecitabine is almost 100% and the half-life is between 0.49 to 0.89 hours [78]

The side effects associated with the use of capecitabine include anemia, diarrhea, nausea, hyperbilirubinemia, fatigue, weakness, abdominal pain, vomiting, and dermatitis [78]

Synthesis

Synthesis of capecitabine (**37**) is outlined in scheme **11**. It is synthesized from 5'-deoxy-5-fluorocytidine (**34**) where hydroxyl groups are first acetylated using acetic anhydride in dry pyridine at 0°C. The acetylated nucleoside (**35**) is then treated with pentylchloroformate at 0°C to yield protected capecitabine (**36**). The compound **36** after deprotection using 1N NaOH afford capecitabine **37** [79]

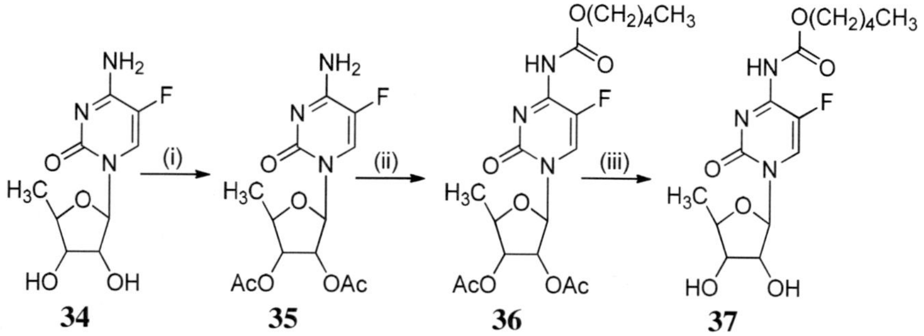

Scheme 11.

Reagent and conditions: (i) Ac$_2$O, dry pyridine, 0 °C, 3 h (ii) pentylchloroformate in toluene, pyridine, CH$_2$Cl$_2$, 0 °C, 1 h (iii) 1N NaOH, CH$_2$Cl$_2$, 0 °C, 1 h.

EMTRICITABINE (FTC)

Emtricitabine or 2',3'-dideoxy-3'-thia-5-fluorocytidine (FTC, **43**) is a nucleoside analog of 5-fluorocytosine with potent antiviral activity against HIV. FTC is also active against HBV.[80a] It was approved by FDA in 2003 for HIV use. [80b,81]. Emtricitabine, in comparison to another well-known antiretroviral drug lamivudine, possesses 4- to 10-fold higher *in vitro* potency against HIV. [82] Emtricitabine was found to display synergism with other anti-retrovirals. However, use of emtricitabine as monotherapy is limited due to its structural similarity to lamivudine and the consequent risk of development of drug resistance. [81]

Emtricitabine is intracellularly phosphorylated to emtricitabine-5'-triphosphate. The triphosphate form then inhibits HIV reverse transcriptase (RT) by competing with the natural substrate deoxycytidine-5'-triphosphate, and/or gets incorporated into growing viral DNA chain resulting in chain termination. In the case of HBV, the emtricitabine-5'-triphosphate inhibits HBV DNA polymerase. [83]

Emtricitabine is usually administered as once a day dose of 200 mg with or without food.[84] Emtricitabine has excellent tolerability and a long intracellular half-life supporting the once-daily dosing. It is rapidly and extensively absorbed following oral administration with peak plasma concentrations occurring at 1–2 hours post-dosing. The mean absolute bioavailability of emtricitabine is 93%

while the mean absolute bioavailability of oral solution is 75%. The biotransformation of emtricitabine includes oxidation of the thiol moiety to form the 3'-sulfoxide diastereomers (~9% of dose) and conjugation with glucuronic acid to form 2'-O-glucuronide (~4% of dose). The plasma half-life of emtricitabine is approximately 10 hours.[81]

The most common adverse reactions of emtricitabine include headache, diarrhea nausea, fatigue, dizziness, depression, insomnia, abnormal dreams, rash, abdominal pain, asthenia, increased cough and rhinitis. [81]

Synthesis

The synthesis of emtricitabine (**43**) has been reported by Schinazi et al [85,86] (scheme **11**). The 5'-butyldipheylsilyl emtricitabine (**41**) was synthesized from protected glyco aldehyde **39**. Reaction of **39** with mercaptoacetic acid in refluxing toluene yielded thialactone **40** in 84% yield. Reduction of **40** using diisobutylaluminum hydride or lithium tri-tert-butoxyaluminum hydride, followed by trapping of the resulting lactol with acetic anhydride, provided **41** as a 2:1 mixture of anomers in 60-80%. Yields. Reaction of this anomeric mixture with silylated 5-fluorocytosine (**4**) and with a Lewis acid led to a mixture of N-glycosylated anomers **42a** and **42b**. However, use of stannic chloride (2 equiv, CH_2Cl_2) at ambient temperature may lead to the exclusive formation of the beta-cytosine adduct **42a**. The adduct **42a** was deblocked using tetrabutylammonium fluoride to give target compound **43** (scheme-12).

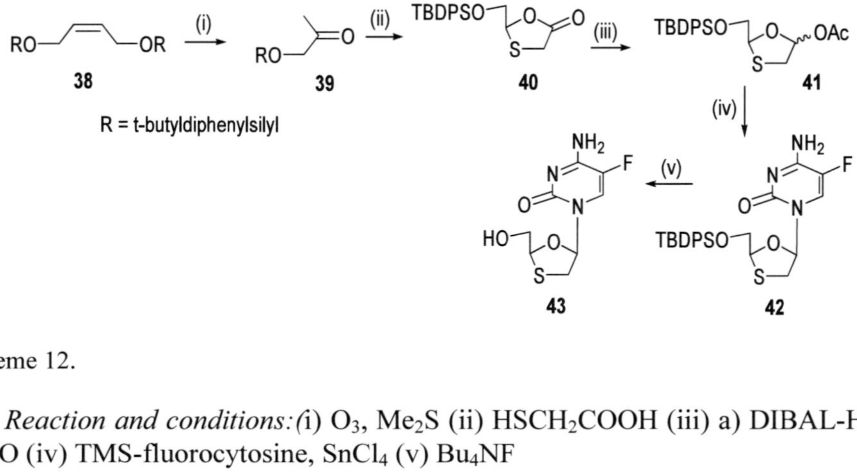

Scheme 12.

Reaction and conditions: (i) O_3, Me_2S (ii) $HSCH_2COOH$ (iii) a) DIBAL-H b) Ac_2O (iv) TMS-fluorocytosine, $SnCl_4$ (v) Bu_4NF

β-D-D4FC AND BETA-L-D4FC

β-D-D4FC

β D-D4FC or *β*-D-2',3'-didehydro-2',3'-dideoxy-5-fluorocytidine (**47**) compound was described in 1986 as a potent and selective anti-HIV agent. *β*-D-d4FC retains activity against HIV isolates resistant to other well-known antiretrovirals such as 3TC and AZT. However, it seems less potent against multi-nucleoside reverse transcriptase inhibitors (NRTI)-resistant viruses, particularly those carrying the Q151M mutation. *β*-D-D4FC is readily converted to its 5'-triphosphate in human peripheral blood mononuclear cells and interacts synergistically with a number of other anti-HIV agents. A phase I clinical study demonstrated that the desired plasma concentrations of *β*-D-D4FC can be easily achieved with an oral dose of 50 mg per day. *β*-D-D4FC may be useful as a once daily component for the treatment of NRTI-experienced patients. In the SCID-hu Thy/Liv mouse model, *β*-D-D4FC reduced the viral load below the detection limit for both the NL4-3 strain designed by deleting a 2 Kb sequence of HIV-1 and 3TC-resistant M184V HIV-1 strains. [87,88]

Beta-L-D4FC (Elvucitabine)

Beta-L-5F-D4C or B-L-2',3'-didehydro-2',3'-dideoxy-5-fluorocytidine (51) is an L-cytosine nucleoside reverse transcriptase inhibitor that has demonstrated potent *in vitro* antiviral activity against HIV, including strains resistant to other NRTIs like its D-counterpart described above. L configuration of this compound provides protection against mitochondrial toxicity often seen with D-nucleosides. Elvucitabine has been demonstrated to have a longer half-life than other approved NRTIs, providing a potential barrier to the emergence of drug resistance in patients who are less than perfectly compliant.[88] Clinical and preclinical data collected to date indicate that elvucitabine can be dosed as a 10-mg pill once daily and can be used in combination therapy.

Synthesis

Beta-D-D4FC (**47**) and beta-L-D4C (**51**) can be synthesized by the coupling reaction of the 5-fluorocytosine (**4**) with beta-D-lactol acetate **44** and beta-L-lactol acetate **48**, in 82% and 66% yields, respectively, (scheme 13). The selenenyl nucleosides **45** and **49** are subjected to oxidative reactions in presence of H_2O_2 to provide the 5'-O-protected 2',3'-dideoxynucleosides **46** and **50,** in 86% and 91% yields, respectively. The deprotection of these compounds by TBAF in THF provides the target nucleosides **47** and **51** [89]

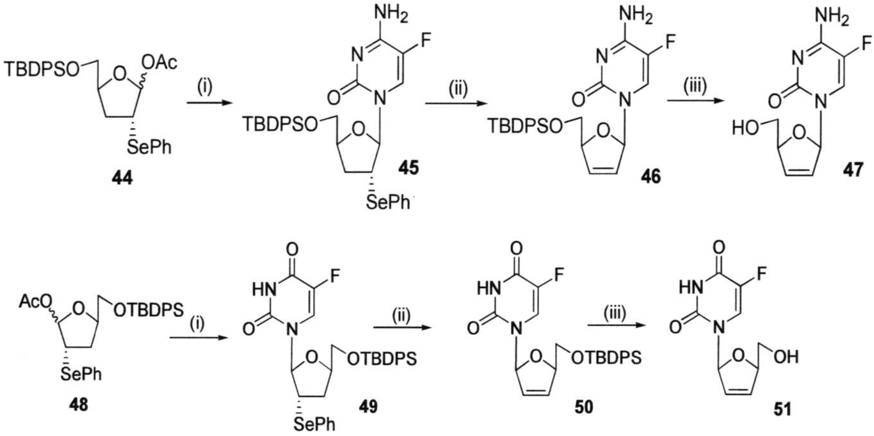

Scheme 13.

Reagent and condition: (i) 5-Fluorocytosine, ammonium sulphate, hexamethyldisilazane, reflux, 2 h, argon atm.; TMSOTf, CH_2Cl_2, 50 °C 15min, r. t. 15 min (ii) CH_2Cl_2, pyridine, H_2O_2, 15 min, 0 °C, 45 min, r. t. 30 min. (iii) 1M tetrabutylammonium fluoride , THF, r.t, 1.5 h. (iv) reagents and conditions as in (i), followed by $SnCl4$ in CH_2Cl_2, r.t. 15 min, 0 °C, 45 min.

ACYCLIC NUCLEOSIDE ANALOGS OF 5-FU

In *in vitro* studies, 5-FU acyclo nucleosides were found to exhibit higher antitumor activity with simultaneously lower toxicity than 5-FU. [90] **Compound 52** was reported to be active against different tumor cell lines *in vitro* and *in vivo* models. In this class of **compound, 53** also exhibited potent *in vitro* (IC_{50} = 9.40 microM) and *in vivo* anticancer activity. [91]

R1 = H or CH₃, R2 = iPr or cyclopentyl

52

53

Kumar and co-workers have also studied a series of acyclic pyrimidine nucleosides possessing a flexible acyclic glycosyl moiety, 1-[(2-hydroxy-1-(hydroxymethyl)ethoxy)methyl], at the N-1 position that can mimic the natural 2-deoxyribosyl moiety and a variety of substituents at the C-5 position of uracil ring including a fluorine. The compounds in which the base moiety was substituted by 5-chloro-, 5-(2-bromovinyl)-, or 5-bromo-6-methyl groups exhibited significant activity against duck-HBV (DHBV), wild-type human HBV (2.2.15 cells), and lamivudine-resistant HBV containing single and double mutations. The compounds 1-[(2-Hydroxy-1-(hydroxymethyl) ethoxy)methyl]-5-fluorouracil (**54**) and 1-[(2-Hydroxy-1-(hydroxymethyl) ethoxy)methyl]-5-fluorocytosine (**55**) with 5-fluoro substituents showed moderate activity against DHBV and human HBV. Compound 55 also displayed some inhibitory activity against hepatitis C virus. The acyclic pyrimidine nucleosides compounds were also investigated for their antiviral activity against West Nile virus, respiratory syncytial virus, and SARS-coronavirus. They were generally inactive in these antiviral assay systems (at concentrations up to 100 μg/mL). Acyclic pyrimidine nucleosides were demonstrated to be non-toxic in host HepG2 and Vero cells, up to the highest concentration tested (>425 μM). [92]

54

55

PEPTIDE DERIVATIVES

5'-Dipeptidyl derivatives of 5-fluoro-2'-deoxyuridine (**56a-d**) have been reported as antibacterial agents. These compounds can be activated by peptide deformylase, which removes the N-terminal formyl group of the dipeptide, to release the active drug FUDR via an intramolecular cyclization reaction. Since the enzyme deformylase is ubiquitous among bacteria but absent in mammalian cells, it was expected that they would have selective activity. However **56a-d** were found to be biologically inactive in *in vitro* assay.[93]

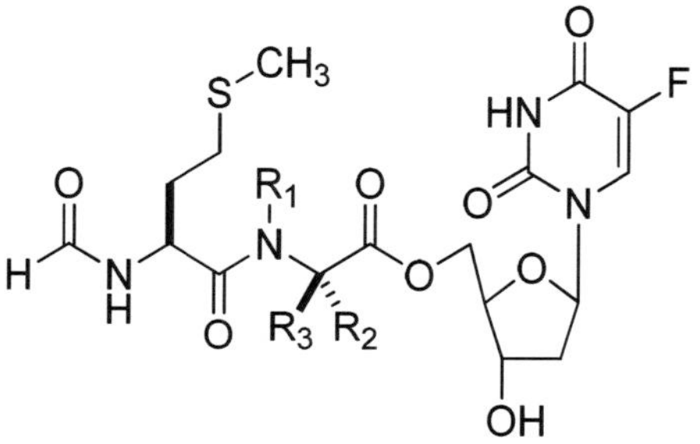

a: R_1-R_2 = $CH_2CH_2CH_2$, R_3= H
b: R_1-R_3 = $CH_2CH_2CH_2$, R_2 = H
c: R_1 = CH_3, R_2 = $CH_2CH(CH_3)_2$, R_3 = H
d: R_1 = H, R_2 = R_3 = CH_3

56

Our group (Shakya et al.) investigated various derivatives of pyrimidine nucleosides containing 5-fluorouracil base as antimycobacterial agents. Compounds **57-61** demonstrated weak to moderate inhibition of various mycobacterial species tested.[94,95]

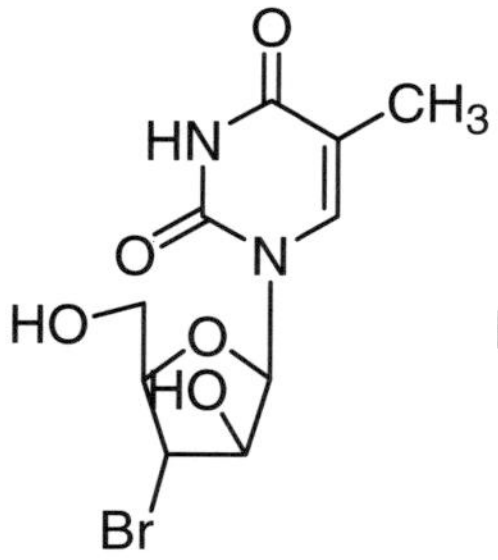

57 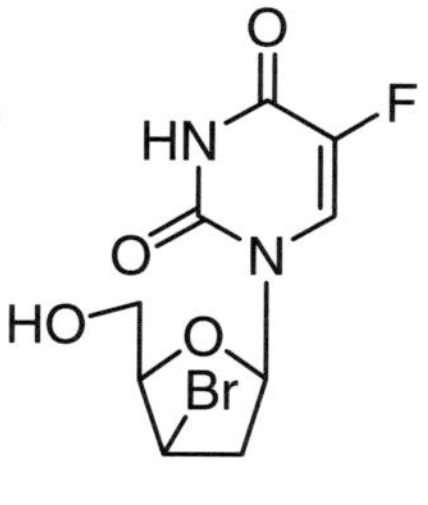   **58** 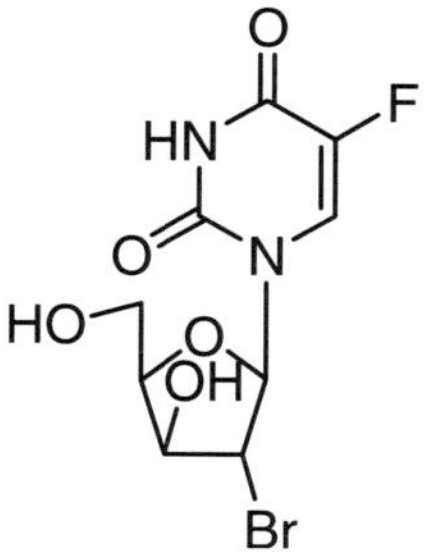   **59**

61

60

CONCLUSION

5-FU and adverse range of its analogs have been of great interest due to their chemotherapeutic properties such as anticancer, antiviral and antibacterial activities. However, many of these drugs/agents suffer from considerable toxicity and pharmacokinetic issues. To overcome these problems, researchers are putting considerable efforts to modify and optimize the chemical entities in 5-FU. 5-FU is mainly used for the treatment of various cancers. On the other hand, its nucleoside analogs have been of interest as antiviral and anticancer agents. 5-FU itself has been evaluated extensively for various diseases/disorders, while its N-substituted derivatives including nucleosides are still being explored. Therefore, broad chemical and biological evaluations are important to obtain their full potential. These efforts will certainly promise effective drug(s) from 5-FU derivatives.

REFERENCES

[1] Cai, T.B.; Tang, X.; Nagorski, J.; Brauschweiger, P.G.; Wang, P.G. *Bioorg. Med. Chem.* 2003, *11,* 4971–4975.

[2] Noordhuis, P.; Holwerda, U.; Van der Wilt, C.L.; Van Groeningen, C.J.; Smid, K.; Meijer, S.; Pinedo H.M.; Peters G.J. *Ann. Oncol.* 2004, *15,* 1025-1032.

[3] Peters, G.J.; Laurensse, E.; Leyva, A et al. *Cancer Res.* 1986, *46,* 20-28.

[4] Miura, K.; Kinouchi, M.; Ishida, K.; Fujibuchi, W.; Naitoh, T.; Ogawa, H.; Ando, T.; Yazaki, N.; Watanabe K.; Haneda, S.; Shibata, C.; Sasaki, I. *Cancers* 2010, *2,* 1717-1730.

[5]   Tian, Z.Y.; Du, G.J.; Xie, S.Q.; Zhao, J.; Gao, W.Y.; Wang C.J. *Molecules.* 2007, *12*, 2450- 2457.

[6]   Zhang, N.; Yin, Y.; Xu, S.J.; Chen, W.S. *Molecules.* 2008, *13*, 1551-1569.

[7]   Ratcliffe, L.; Beadsworth, M.B.; Pennell, A.; Phillips, M.; Vilar, F.J. Managing hepatitis B/HIV co-infected: adding entecavir to truvada (tenofovirdisoproxil/ emtricitabine) experienced patients. AIDS. 2011, 25 (8), 1051-1056.

[8]   Heidelberger, C.; Chaudhuri, N.K.; Danneberg, P.; Mooren, D.; Griesbach, L.; Duschinsky, R.; Schnitzer, R.J.; Pleven, E.; Scheiner, J. *Nature* 1957, *179*, 663–666.

[9]   Rutman, R.J.; Cantarow, A.; Paschkis, K.E. *J. Biol. Chem.* 1954, *210*, 321–329.

[10]   Rutman, R. J.; Cantarow, A.; Paschkis, K. E. *Cancer Res.* 1954, *14*, 119-123.

[11]   Douillard, J. Y.; Cunningham, D.; Roth, A. D.; Navarro, M.; James, R. D.; Karasek, P.; Jandik, P.; Iveson, T.; Carmichael, J.; Alakl, M.; Gruia, G.; Awad, L.; Rougier, P. *Lancet* 2000, *355*, 1041-1047.

[12]   Chu, E.; Mota, A.C.; Fogarasi MC (2001) Pharmacology of cancer chemotherapy. In: DeVita VT, Hellman S, Rosenberg SA (Eds) Cancer: principles and practice of oncology 6th edn. Lippincott Williams and Wilkins, Philadelphia, pp 388.

[13]   Cunningham, D.; James, R. D. *Eur. J. Cancer* 2001, *37*, 826-834.

[14]   Spears, C.P.; Shani, J.; Shahinian, A.H et al. *Mol. Pharmacol.* 1984, 27, 302–307.

[15]   Goshal, K.; Jacob, S.T. *Biochem. Pharmacol.* 1997, *53*, 1569–1575.

[16]   Major, P.P.; Egan, E.; Herrick, D.; Kufe, D.W. *Cancer. Res.* 1982, *42*, 3005 – 3009.

[17]   Sawyer, R.C.; Stolfi, R.L.; Martin, D.S.; Spiegelman, S. *Cancer. Res.* 1984, *44*, 1847-1851.

[18]   Peters G.J; Ko¨ hne CH. Fluoropyrimidines as antifolate drugs. In Jackman J.L. (ed.): *Antifolate Drugs in Cancer Therapy.* Totowa, NJ: Humana Press 1999; 101-145.

[19]   Longley, D.B.; Harkin, D.P.; Johnston, P.G. *Nat. Rev. Cancer.* 2003, *3*, 330-338.

[20]   20.   Iyer, L.; Ratain, M.J. *Cancer. Invest.* 1999, *17*, 494-506.

[21]   Package insertGensiaSicor Pharmaceutical. Available from http://patient. cancerconsultants.com/druginserts/Fluorouracil.pdf.Accessed on Jan 7, 2012.

[22] Hsiao, H.H.; Yang, M.Y.; Chang, J.G.; Liu, Y.C.; Liu, T.C.; Chang, C.S.; Chen, T.P.; Lin, S.F. *Cancer Chemother. Pharmacol.* 2004, *53*, 445-451.

[23] Joulia, J.M.; Pinguet, F.; Ychou, M.; Duffour, J.; Astre, C.; Bressolle, F. *Eur. J. Cancer.* 1999, *35*, 296-301.

[24] Houghton, J.A.; Houghton, P.J.; Wooten, R.S. *Cancer Res.* 1979, *39*, 2406–2413.

[25] Schuetz, J.D.; Wallace, H.J.; Diasio, R.B.*Cancer Res.* 1984, *44*, 1358–1363.

[26] Muneoka, K.; Shirai, Y.; Yokoyama, N.; Wakai, T.; Hatakeyama, K. *Int. J. Clin. Oncol.* 2005, *10*, 441-443.

[27] Barton, D.H.; Hesse, R.H.; Pechet, M.M. et al. *Org Chem.* 1972, *37*, 329-330.

[28] Duschchinsky, R.; Pleven, E.; Heidelberger, C. *J. Am. Chem. Soc.* 1957, *79*, 4559-4560.

[29] Heidelberger, C.; Griesbach, L.; Montag, B.J.; Mooren, D.; Cruz, O.; Schnitzer, R.J et al. *Cancer Research.* 1958, *18*, 305-317.

[30] Bennett, J. E.; Dismukes, W. E.; Duma, R. J.; Medoff, G.; Sande, M.A.; Gallis, H et al. *New Eng. J. Med.* 1979, 301, 126-131.

[31] Patel, R. *Mayo Clinic Proceedings.* 1998, 73, 1205-1225.

[32] Grunberg, E.; Titsworth, E.; Bennett,M. (1963). *Antimicrob.Agents Chemother.* 1963, *3*, 566-568.

[33] Tassel, D.; Madoff, M.A. *J. Am. Med. Asso.* 1968, *201*, 830-832.

[34] Benson, J. M.; Nahata, M. C. *Clinical Pharmacy.* 1988, *7*, 424-438.

[35] Bennet, J.E. *Ann. Inter. Med.*1977, *86*, 319-321.

[36] Lefrock, J.L.; Smith, B.R. *Am. Fam. Physician.* 1984, *30*, 162-167.

[37] Vermes, A.; Guchelaar, H.J.; Dankert, J. *J. Antimicrob. Chemother.* 2000, *46*, 171-179.

[38] Cutler, R. E.; Blair, A. D.; Kelly, M. R. *Clin. Pharmacol.ther.* 1978, *24*, 333-342.

[39] Vermes, A.; vandersijs, I. H.; Guchelaar, H. J. *Chemotherapy.* 2000, *46*, 86-94.

[40] Kauffman, C.A.; Frame, P. T. *Antimicrob. Agents Chemother.*1977, *11*, 244-247.

[41] Finch, R. E.; Bending, M.R.; Lant, A. F. *Br. J. Clin. Pharmacol.* 1979, *7*, 613-617.

[42] Morris, J.; Robins, S. R. *J. Chem. Soc.; Chem. Commun.*; 1972, 18-19.

[43] Rathod, P.K.; Khatri, A.; Hubbert, T.; Milhous, WK.*Antimicrob Agents Chemother.* 1989, *33*, 1090-1094.

[44] Muregi, F.W.; Kano, S.; Kino, H.; Ishih, A.*ExpParasitol.* 2009, *121,* 376-380.

[45] Rathod, P.K.; Reyes, P. *J Biol Chem.* 1998, *258,* 2852-2855.

[46] Heidelberger, C.; Danenberg, P. V.; Moran, R.G. *Adv. Enzymol.*1983, *119,*54- 57.

[47] Chaudhuri, N.K.; Montag, B.J.; Heidelberger, C. Cancer Res. 1958, 18, (3), 318-328.

[48] Miyazaki, N.; Tabata, Y.*J. Nanosci. Nanotechnol.* 2009, *9,* 4797-4804.

[49] Maehara, Y.; Anai, H.; Kusumoto, H.; Kusumoto, T.; Sugimachi, K. *Dis Colon Rectum.*1988, 31 (1), 62-67.

[50] Gröhn, P.; Heinonen, E.; Kumpulainen, E.; Länsimies, H.; Lantto, A.; Salmi, R.; Pyrhönen, S.; Numminen, S. *Am J ClinOncol.* 1990, 13 (6), 477-479.

[51] Sakamoto, J.; Hamada, C.; Rahmanm, M.; Kodaira, S.; Ito, K.; Nakazato, H.; Ohashi, Y.; Yasutomi, M. *Jpn J ClinOncol.* 2005, *35,* 536-544.

[52] Matsumoto, S.; Nishizawa, S.; Murakami, M.; Noma, S.; Sano, A.; Kuroda, Y. *Neuroradiology.* 1995, *37,* 649-652.

[53] Ozaki, S. *Medicinal Research Reviews.* 1996, 16 (1), 51-86 and reference therein. John Wiley& Sons, Inc. Available from http://www.scribd.com/doc/38723284/Synthesis-and-Antitumor-Activity-of-5-Fluorouracil-Derivatives, Accessed on Jan 7, 2012.

[54] Kametani, T.; Kigasawa, K.; Hiiragi, M.; Wakisaka, K.; Haga, S.; Nagamatsu, Y.; Sugi, H.; Fukawa, K.; Irino, O.; Yamamoto, T.; Nishimura, N.; Taguchi, A.; Okada, T.; Nakayama, M. *J. Med. Chem.* 1980, 23 (12), 1324-1329.

[55] Liu, C.; Liu, D.; Bai, F, Zhang, J.; Zhang, N. *Drug Delivery* 2010, 17(5), 352-363.

[56] Zhang, X.; Zhong, J. L.; Liu, W.; Gao, Z.; Xue, X.; Yue, P.; Wang, L.; Zhao, C.; Xu, W.; Qu, X. *Cancer Chemother Pharmacol.* 2010, 66 (1), 11-19.

[57] Sun, W.; Zhang, N.; Li, A.; Zou, W.; Xu, W. 2008, *Int. J. Pharm.353,* 243–250.

[58] Yasumoto, M.; Yamawaki, I.; Marunaka, T.; Hashimoto, S. *J. Med. Chem.* 1978, 21 (8), 738-41.

[59] Tanaka, F. *Surg Today.* 2007, 37 (11), 923-943.

[60] Tanaka, F.; Fukuse, T.; Wada, H.; Fukushima, M. *Curr. Pharm. Biotechnol.* 2000, *1* (2), 137-164.

[61] Kametani, T.; Kigasawa, K.; Hiragi, M.; Wakisaka, K.; Kusama, O.; Kawasaki, K.; Sugi, H. *J. Hetrocyclic Chem.* 1977, 14. 473-474.

[62] Ardalan, B.; Lima, M. A. *J. Cancer Res. Clin .Oncol.* 2004, 130 (10), 561-566.

[63] Power, D. G.; Kemeny, N. E. *Mol Cancer Ther.* 2009, 8 (5), 1015-1025.

[64] Available from http://www.drugbank.ca/drugs/DB00322 (Accessed in April 2012)

[65] Dawson, W.H. and Dunlap, R.B. *Journal of labelled Compounds and Radiopharmceuticals.* 1979, Vol. XVI, (2), 335-343.

[66] Beumer, J, H.; Eiseman, J. L.; Parise, R, A.; Joseph, E.; Holleran, J. L.; Covey, J. M.; Egorin, M. J.*Clin Cancer Res.* 2006, 12 (24), 7483-7491.

[67] Beumer, J. H.; Parise, R. A.; Newman, E. M.; Doroshow, J. H.; Synold, T. W.; Lenz, H. J.; Egorin, M. *J Cancer ChemotherPharmacol.* 2008, 62 (2), 363-368.

[68] Cai, F.F.; Kohler, C.; Zhang, B.; Wang, M.H.; Chen, W.J.; Zhong, X.Y. *Int J Mol Sci.* 2011, 12 (7), 4465-4487. 79. 63.

[69] (a) Tunio, M.A.; Hashmi, A.; Shoaib, M. REPORT: *Pak J Pharm Sci.* 2012, *25* (1), 277-281 (b) Beumer J. H.; Eiseman, J. L.;, Parise, R. A.; Joseph, E.; Holleran, J. L.; Covey, J.M.; Egorin, M. *J. Clin Cancer Res.* 2006, 12, 7483-7491.

[70] Duschinsky, R.; Gabriel, T.; Hoffer, M.; Berger, J.; Titsworth, E.; Grunberg, E.; Burchenal, J.H.; Fox, J.J. *J. Med. Chem.* 1966, 9 (4), 566-572.

[71] Cook, A. F.; Holman, M. J.; Kramer, M. J.; Trown, P. W. *J Med Chem.* 1979, *22* (11), 1330-1335.

[72] Maeda, H.; Kusuhara, T.; Tsuhako, M.; Nakayama, H. *Chem Pharm Bull.* 2011, *59* (12), 1447-1451.

[73] Yamashita, T.; Yamashita, H.; Itoh, Y.; Karamatsu, S.; Itoh, K.; Hara, Y.; Ando, Y.; Sugiura, H.; Kuzushima, T.; Toyama, T.; Iwata, H.; Kobayashi, S.; Iwase, H. *Breast Cancer.* 2006, *13*(4), 334-339.

[74] Yoshikawa, T.; Tsuburaya, A.; Shimada, K.; Sato, A.; Takahashi, M.; Koizumi, W.; Yoshizawa, Y.; Nabeshima, K.; Kimura, M.; Hataya, K.; Kobayashi, O. *Gastric Cancer.* 2009, *12*(4), 212-218.

[75] Bajetta, E.; Di, Bartolomeo, M.; Somma, L.; Del, Vecchio, M.; Artale, S.; Zunino, F.; Bignami, P.; Magnani, E.; Buzzoni, R. *Eur J Cancer.* 1997, 33 (4), 687-690.

[76] Van, Der, Heyden, S. A.; Highley, M. S.; De, Bruijn, E. A.; Tjaden, U. R.; Reeuwijk, H. J.; Van, Slooten, H.; Van, Oosterom, A. T.; Maes, R. *Br. J. ClinPharmacol.* 1999 ,47 (4), 351-356.

[77]   Ebi, H.; Sigeoka, Y.; Saeki, T.; Kawada, K.; Igarashi, T.; Usubuchi, N.; Ueda, R.; Sasaki, Y.; Minami, H. *Cancer Chemother Pharmacol.* 2005, 56 (2), 205-211.

[78]   Hirsch, B.R.; Zafar, S.Y. *Cancer Manag Res.* 2011, *3*, 79-89.

[79]   Arasaki, M.; Ishitsuka, H.; Kuruma, I; Miwa, M.; Murasaki, C.; Shimma, N.; Umeda, I. N-4-(Substituted-oxycarbonyl)-5'-deoxy-5-fluorocytidine compounds, compositions and methods of using the same. U. S. Patent no. 5,472,949. Date of patent Dec 5, 1995.

[80]   (a) Nelson, M; Schiavone, M. Int J ClinPract, 2004, 58, 5, 504–510. (b) De, Clercq, E. *Int J Antimicrob Agents.* 2009, 33 (4), 307-320.

[81]   Gilead Sciences. Emtriva (emtricitabine) capsules prescribing information. Available at http://www.gilead.com/pdf/emtriva_pi.pdf. Accessed on Jan 5, 2012.

[82]   De, Clercq, E.*J Med Chem.* 2005, 48 (5), 1297-1313.

[83]   Gish, R, G.; Leung, N. W.; Wright, T. L.; Trinh, H.; Lang, W.; Kessler, H. A.; Fang, L.; Wang, L. H.; Delehanty, J.; Rigney, A.; Mondou, E.; Snow, A.; Rousseau, F. *Antimicrob Agents Chemother.* 2002, 46 (6), 1734-1740.

[84]   Available   from   http://www.ncbi.nlm.nih.gov/pubmedhealth/ PMH0000248/. Accessed on Jan 3, 2012.

[85]   Woo-Baeg Choi, W.B.; Wilson, L.J.; Yeola, S.; Liotta, D. C. *J. Am. Chem. SOC.* 1991, *113,* 9377-9379

[86]   Schinazi R.F.; Boudinot, F.D.; Ibrahim, S.S.; Manning, C.; McClure H.M.; Liotta, D.C. *Antimicrob Agents Chemother.* 1992, 36 (11), 2432-8.

[87]   De, Clercq, E. *J Med Chem.* 2005, 48 (5), 1297-1313.

[88]   De, Clercq, E. Emerging antiviral drugs. *Expert Opin Emerg Drugs.* 2008, 13 (3), 393-416.

[89]   Shi J.; McAtee J.J.; SchlueterWirtz S.; Tharnish, P.; Juodawlkis, A.; Liotta, D.C.; Schinazi, R.F. *J. Med. Chem.* 1999, 42 (5), 859-867.

[90]   Ajmera, S. Bapat, A.R.; Stephanian, E.; Danenberg, P.V. *J. Med. Chem.;* 1988, *31,* 1094-1098.

[91]   Marchal, J. A.; Nunez; M. C.; Aranega, A.; Gallo, M. A.; Espinosa, A.; Campos, J. M. *Curr Med Chem.* 2009, 16 (9), 1166-1183.

[92]   Kumar. R.; Semaine, W.; Johar, M.; Tyrrell, D.L.; Agrawal, B. *J Med Chem.* 2006, 49 (12), 3693-3700.

[93]   Wei, Y.; Pei, D. *Bioorg. Med. Chem. Lett.* 2000, 10 (10), 1073-1076.

[94]   Shakya, N.; Srivastav, N.C.; Desroches, N.; Agrawal, B.; Kunimoto, D.Y.; Kumar, R.*J. Med. Chem.* 2010, 53 (10), 4130-4140.

[95]   Johar, M.; Manning, T.; Kunimoto, D. Y.; Kumar, R. *Bioorg Med Chem.* 2005 13 (24), 6663-6671.

In: Fluorouracil
Editors: A. Longinho and S. Dobreiro

ISBN: 978-1-62081-970-8
© 2012 Nova Science Publishers, Inc.

Chapter III

5-FLUOROURACIL AND ITS IMMUNOTOXICITY: A CLINICAL AND EXPERIMENTAL APPROACH

*Adriana Andrade Carvalho[1] and Daniel Pereira Bezerra[2],**
[1]School of Pharmacy, Federal University of Sergipe,
Lagarto, Sergipe, Brazil
[2]Department of Physiology, Federal University of Sergipe,
São Cristóvão, Sergipe, Brazil

ABSTRACT

5-Fluorouracil (5-FU), a fluorinated pyrimidine that belongs to the group of antimetabolites, has become a component of the standard therapy for a variety of solid tumors, including gastrointestinal, head and neck, and breast cancers. The common clinical toxicity of 5-FU is affect the *rapidly dividing tissues* such as the bone marrow hematopoietic cells, which induces an important immunosuppression that potentially causes infection easily and reduced anticancer immunity. In this chapter, the clinical immunological effects of 5-FU, as well as experimental models used to assess and identify new compounds to treat 5-FU-induced immunotoxicity, were summarized. Experimentally, peripheral hematological and bone marrow analysis, cytokines quantification, and histological examination of the thymus, spleen,

---

* Correspondence author: Prof. Dr. Daniel Pereira Bezerra, Federal University of Sergipe, Department of Physiology, Av. Marechal Rondon, Jardim Rosa Elze, 49100-000, São Cristovão, Sergipe, Brazil. Phone + 55 79 2105 6644, E-mail: danielpbezerra@gmail.com.

and lymphoid organs have been used to assess the immunosuppression in 5-FU-treated animals. Different compounds have been described in literature as agents able to prevent/reduce 5-FU-induced immunotoxicity, including chitosans and polysaccharides. In summary, these data should be used to establish new directions and new goals in future research.

Keywords: 5-fluorouracil, side effects, immunotoxicity

INTRODUCTION

The fluoropyrimidine 5-fluorouracil (5-FU), an antimetabolite drug, works by being incorporated into the RNA and DNA and by the inhibition of the nucleotide synthetic enzyme thymidylate synthase. It is widely used in the treatment of a range of cancers, including gastrointestinal, head and neck, and breast cancers (Malet-Martino and Martino, 2002; Longley et al., 2003). However, an important clinical side effect of 5-FU is that it affects the normal proliferating tissue cells such as bone marrow cells (Ohta et al., 1980; Malet-Martino and Martino, 2002).

Bone marrow is the manufacturing center for blood cells; the suppression of bone marrow activity, sometimes called myelotoxicity or myelosuppression, causes a deficiency of blood cells. Three different kinds of blood cells are produced in the body's bone marrow: red blood cells, white blood cells, and platelets (Tavassoli, 1991; Ogawa, 1993; Flemming and Weissman, 1995). Myelosuppression can result in the decrease in one, two or all three types of blood cells. When chemotherapy induces the reduction of red blood cells, white blood cells, and platelet numbers, the result is anemia, leukopenia/leukocytopenia, and thrombocytopenia, respectively. If an individual experiences a drop in all three types of blood cells, the condition is called pancytopenia. All forms of myelosuppression are frequent and potentially seriously complicate 5-FU administration (Macdonald et al., 1999; Ho et al., 2011). The molecular machinery governing 5-FU-mediated myelotoxicity is obscure; however, at least in part, the oxidative stress in bone marrow induced by 5-FU seems to be involved (Numazawa et al., 2011).

In particular, lowered production of white blood cells reduces the activation or efficacy of the immune system. This unwanted effect results in increased susceptibility to pathogens, such as bacteria and virus, and reduces the anticancer immunity. As a result, fever and chills are the most common side effect of reduced white blood cells. Signs of infection may also be present, including swelling, redness or an area that is warm to the touch. Other common side effects include diarrhea and rash (Macdonald et al., 1999; Choi et al., 2003).

These therapeutics-derived poor conditions can be major disruptions to effective treatment with optimal therapeutic dosages or for sufficient therapeutic periods; therefore, they are also main factors lowering the quality of life for cancer patients. Several alternative strategies have been tried, as well as management with many Colony Stimulating Factors (CSFs) (Pettengell et al., 1992; Ozer et al., 2000; Dale, 2002). However, their lower efficiency and clinical limitations still require novel agents and therapeutics to treat 5-FU-induced immunotoxicity. In this chapter, the clinical immunological effects of 5-FU, as well as experimental models used to assess and identify new compounds to treat 5-FU-induced immunotoxicity, were summarized. These data should be used to establish new directions and new goals in future research.

5-FU-INDUCED IMMUNOTOXICITY IN CLINICAL THERAPY

The side effects of 5-FU are schedule-dependent. For the bolus regimen, toxicities include myelosuppression, oral mucositis, and gastrointestinal disturbances (diarrhea, nausea, and vomiting). For the continuous regimen, toxic reactions include the hand-foot syndrome (HFS, i.e., dermal pain in hands and feet), which was observed in many cases, and a lower frequency of hematologic and gastrointestinal toxicity. Cardiotoxicity and neurotoxicity may be observed during treatment with 5-FU (2%-5% of cases), but symptoms disappear on stopping treatment, and resumption of treatment with a lower dose is generally well tolerated (Macdonald et al., 1999; Malet-Martino and Martino, 2002; Katzung, 2003).

The immunosuppressive activity of 5-FU is a serious and paradoxical side effect from the aspect of its therapeutic efficacy. The immunosuppression reduces the therapeutic effect of 5-FU because it causes not only damage in the immunological defense function toward infections but also a dysfunction of immunological resistance against the tumor (Mitchell et al., 1990; Kimura and Okuda, 1999a; Kobayashi et al., 2006).

Treatment by continuous i.v. infusion of 5-FU presents advantages compared with treatment by bolus i.v. with respect to both efficacy and toxicity, although the mean survival rate is no better. On the other hand, treatment by continuous i.v. infusion showed a high cost, and the added risks mean that it is used relatively infrequently; thus, i.v. bolus remains the main treatment (Malet-Martino and Martino, 2002). Leucovorin (LV, folinic acid, 5-formyl tetrahydrofolate), by ensuring the thymidylate synthase-5-fluorodeoxyuridine monophosphate-folate complex formation, is commonly supplemented as a biomodulator in 5-FU regimens. Experimental and clinical experiences suggest that a longer and sustained exposure to 5-FU plasma concentration through continuous infusion, together with LV, results in superior tumor response and less toxicity (Poon et al., 1991; Buroker et al., 1994; Yeh et al., 2000a, 200b).

The maximum tolerated doses for 5-FU in protracted 28-day continuous infusion and in weekly high-dose 5-FU/LV 24 h continuous infusion protocols were determined to be 450 mg/m^2/day and 2600 mg/m^2/24 h/week, respectively (Spicer et al., 1988; Ardalan et al., 1991). Other protocols, sometimes with LV dosage reduction, have been adopted with satisfactory responses without calcite precipitation (Yeh and Cheng, 1994; Yeh et al., 1997). Moreover, different research groups have evaluated a 48 h continuous infusion 5-FU schedule. However, this regimen resulted in variable outcomes depending on the 5-FU dosage (2000-4000 mg/m^2/48 h), administration frequency (weekly vs. bimonthly), presence of LV modulation (with vs. without), LV dosage (0-500 mg/m^2/day), and route of LV administration (oral vs. intravenous) (Shah et al., 1985; Diaz-Rubio et al., 1990; Aranda et al., 1995, 1996, 1998 ; De Gramont et al., 1997, 1998; Beerblock et al., 1997).

The majority of studies observe a significant association between genetic variants in dihydropyrimidine dehydrogenase (DPD) gene (DPYD) and severe 5-FU-related toxicities. There are laboratory tests to determine the relative activity of the DPD enzyme. DPD deficiency, a pharmacogenetic syndrome leading to partial or total loss of ability to detoxify 5-FU in the liver, is strongly associated with increased risk of severe/lethal toxicities with 5-FU (Ciccolini et al., 2010; Amstutz et al., 2011).

EXPERIMENTAL MODELS USED TO ASSESS THE 5-FU-INDUCED IMMUNOTOXICITY

One available model to study the immune stimulatory effect of drugs on myelosuppression caused by 5-FU is using animal models after a single exposition of 5-FU. The animals (usually male or female mice, $n = 6\text{-}10$, 10-12 weeks of age, 20-30 g; or rats, 12-14 weeks of age, 150-250 g) can be treated with 5-FU acutely for 1 day (with a usual dose of 100 mg/kg, i.p.) or sub-chronically for 5-10 consecutive days (with a usual dose of 10-25 mg/kg, i.p.). The test substance can be administered before or together with 5-FU treatment at different doses or protocols. In classical protocols, treatment can be performed in healthy or tumor-bearing animals (Wang et al., 1992; Konishi et al., 1996, 2002; Kimura and Okuda, 1999a, 1999b; Assef et al., 2002; Djazayeri et al., 2005; Choi et al., 2007; Bezerra et al., 2006, 2008a, 2008b; Gonzaga et al., 2009; Zheng et al., 2010; Chen et al., 2010; Asanuma et al., 2010; Magalhães et al., 2011a). Briefly, 24-48 hours after the end of treatment, the assessment of the immunological system can be performed as described below.

Hematological analysis - For the hematological analysis, an aliquot of blood from each animal is mixed with ethylenediaminetetraacetic acid (EDTA), and hematological parameters are determined by standard manual procedures using light microscopy or by automated system.

Cytokines quantification - Plasma is obtained after centrifugation of blood for 5 minutes at 14,000 G. Plasma samples are diluted four-fold with PBS and assayed by enzyme-linked immunosorbent assay (ELISA). This assay can be used to measure: inflammatory cytokines, like IL-1, that can be found as a membrane-bound protein α or in a soluble secreted form β, and participate in paracrine and autocrine signaling; IL-6 also known as B-cell differentiation factor, T-cell differentiation factor, hybridoma/plasmacytoma growth factor, and hepatocyte stimulating factor; IL-2, a cytokine secreted by T-cells to stimulate T-cell proliferation and facilitate the development of cell-mediated immunity; IFN-γ, a cytokine secreted by NK cells and CD4 and CD8 T-cell lymphocytes, that activates macrophages (Mph) and is associated with the development of strong cellular immunity, both of which play an important role in fighting viral infection and in antitumor effects (Mosmann and Sad, 1996; Young and Hardy, 1995).

Bone marrow analysis - After the sacrifice of the animals, the bone marrow cells from control and experimental mice are flushed from the femurs and tibias of each mouse using a-minimal essential medium (a-MEM) containing 5% fetal calf serum (FCS). A single-cell suspension is obtained by passing the bone marrow cell suspension through a 25-gauge needle several times before pelleting the cells using a centrifuge (500 G for 10 minutes) and resuspending the cells in fresh a-MEM medium (Wang et al., 1991; Timeus et al., 2003). The bone marrow cells recovered from the mice are counted and assayed for cell cycle by flow cytometry to estimate the percentage of cells arrested in G_0/G_1 phase. Then, the cells (10^5 cells) are plated in agarose cultures with or without an addition of 10% (v/v) mouse lung conditioned medium (LCM). After 7-9 days of incubation, the total number of colonies (> 100 cells) is counted using an inverted microscope. The morphology of the colony is determined in situ after fixation with 5% glutaraldehyde, dehydration with methanol, and staining with hematoxylin. Identifiable colonies are microscopically classified as either purely myeloid (colony-forming unit granulocyte-macrophage [CFC-GM]) or erythroid cells (CFC-E) (Wang et al., 1991; Timeus et al., 2003; Lorenz et al., 2010).

Morphological and histological analysis - Histological examination of the bone marrow, thymus, spleen, and lymphoid organs has been used to assess the immunosuppression in 5-FU-treated animals. The organs are weighed, and the ratios of these organ weights to the body weight (relative weight) are calculated based on the final body weight. For the histopathological evaluation, the organs are fixed in 10% neutral buffered formalin. The femur must be decalcified using Plank-Rychlo solution (Shibata et al., 2000). After fixation, sections (3-5 μm) of the organs are prepared, and slides are mounted for histological analysis. Hematoxylin and eosin (HE) stained specimens are prepared and subjected to microscopic observation to determine changes that may indicate a possible immunostimulatory effect (Asanuma et al., 2010; Wang et al., 1992).

EXPERIMENTAL SUBSTANCES ABLE TO PREVENT/REDUCE THE 5-FU-INDUCED IMMUNOTOXICITY

Different compounds have been tested as agents able to prevent/reduce the 5-FU-induced immunotoxicity, including chitosans and polysaccharides. They are described below.

Chitosan - Chitosan is a polymer with a molecular weight of about 1000 kDa that contains more than 5,000 glucosamine units. It is a natural product obtained by deacetylation of its parent polymer chitin, a polysaccharide widely distributed in nature (e.g., crustaceans, insects and certain fungi) (Dasha et al., 2011; Kimura, 2003). Kimura and Okuda (1999a) demonstrated that Chitosan has an antitumor activity in Sarcoma 180-bearing mice, with an abolition of reduction of blood leukocyte number caused by 5-FU administration. Furthermore, the association of 5-FU plus Chitosan also prevented the reduction of spleen weight induced by 5-FU in Sarcoma 180-bearing mice. Chitosan also inhibits the reduction of lymphocyte, CD8$^+$ T-cell, and NK cell numbers induced by 5-FU in C57BL/6 mice (Kimura and Okuda, 1999a), which demonstrates the immunoprotective proprieties of Chitosan on immunosuppression induced by 5-FU.

Common Carp Extract (Cyprinus carpio L.) - Common carp (*Cyprinus carpio* L.) is one of the most important fish cultured worldwide, of which more than 2.7 million tons were produced in the year 2000 (Rairakhwada et al., 2007). Carp has been used in Korea, China and Japan as a health food source. Kimura and Okuda (1999b) show that oral administration of carp extract has significant antitumor activity; however, 5-FU plus carp extract inhibited tumor growth similarly to 5-FU alone. It was also observed that the reduction of leukocyte number caused by 5-FU administration was significantly inhibited by the oral administration of carp extract, and the reduction of spleen weight induced by 5-FU was slightly inhibited by the concomitant oral administration of carp extract (Kimura, 2003; Kimura and Okuda, 1999b).

Chinese Herbal Formula, Bing De Ling - Bing De Ling is a Chinese herbal mixture formulated to boost the body's immune responses and resistance to viral infection and to preserve its homeostatic balance. Most commonly prescribed in complementary medical settings against common colds, influenza, chronic fatigue syndrome, herpes simplex, herpes zoster, and other viral disorders, Bing De Ling use is based on the modern knowledge of its ingredients' biochemical activities and traditional Chinese herbal formulatory principles to boost the body's immune system (Niu et al., 2000). Bing De Ling solution consists of astragalus root (*Astragalus membranaceus*), rhubarb root (*Rheum palmatum*), white atractylodes (*Atractylodes macrocephala*), isatis root (*Isatis tinctoria*), scutilliar root (*Scutellaria baicalensis*), dogberry (*Cormus officinalis*), and shield fern root (*Dryopnteris erassirhizoma*) at a concentration of 0.121 g/ml of water (Xu et al., 2005). A study performed by Niu et al. (2000) suggests that Bing De Ling potentiates up-regulation of immune activity in a murine model. They showed a two-fold to four-fold elevation of *ex vivo* IL-2 and IFN-γ production. Bing De Ling treatment has also stimulated antitumor cytotoxic activity of NK cells, LAK cells, and Mph obtained from Bing De Ling-treated mice. As these results encompass both primary killing of tumor cells and production of secondary cytokine messengers, stimulation of the network of immunologic responses is implied. Xu et al. (2005) observed that Bing De Ling enhances the antitumor effect and survival rates of 5-FU and inhibits the 5-FU-induced IL-6 up-regulation (Xu et al., 2005).

α-(1-4)-glucan–β-(1-6)-glucan-protein complex polysaccharide - *Agaricus blazei* Murill, popularly known as ''Cogumelo do Sol'', is a native mushroom of Brazil, found particularly in the state of São Paulo. Since 1965, the strains have been exported to Japan, where this mushroom has become popularly known as ''Himematsutake'' or ''Kawarihara-take'' (Gonzaga et al., 2009). The beneficial effects of edible and medicinal mushrooms have long been recognized, and mushrooms have become popular as ordinary foods and dietary supplements worldwide (Lee et al., 2008). The antimutagenic, antioxidant, immunostimulatory and antitumorigenic activities of this Brazilian mushroom have been observed in previous works. Gonzaga et al. (2009) investigated the effects of α-(1-4)-glucan–β-(1-6)-glucan-protein complex polysaccharide from *A. blazei* Murill alone and

associated with 5-FU in experimental models. Using Swiss mice bearing Sarcoma 180, the polysaccharide had antitumor activity and was also able to increase the response elicited by 5-FU. The animals treated with 5-FU presented leukopenia, which was prevented by the association with the polysaccharide, indicating a protective effect of the polysaccharide against delayed hematopoietic depression induced by 5-FU. The combination of the polysaccharide and 5-FU did not lead to substantial changes in biochemical, hematological, and histopathological parameters.

Polysaccharide of black soybean (PSBS) - Soybean [*Glycine max* (L.) Merr.] is nutritionally attractive in that it has different seed coat colors, including black, brown, red, green, and yellow. In particular, black soybeans containing black seed coats have been a widely used crop for many years due to their dietary health benefits and use in folk medicine (Lee and Cho, 2012). In traditional Chinese medicine, black soybean has been used for detoxification, as an anti-inflammatory, and to improve the blood. Soybean has been reported to possess many properties, including immune modulation (Gladysheva et al., 2001), inhibition of carcinogenesis (Suzuki et al., 2002), antioxidation (Minemoto et al., 2002), and a cholesterol lowering effect (Kerckhoffs et al., 2002). Liao et al. (2005) tested the reconstitution effect of PSBS on myelosuppression induced by 5-FU using ICR mice. They found that the baseline leukocyte count of ICR mice in untreated control and PSBS-treated groups were similar, but 5-FU caused apparent myelosuppression. Treatment with PSBS for 5 days not only reduced the degree of leukopenia caused by 5-FU but also shortened the recovery time of leukocyte counts. After 5-FU treatment, the colony forming unit-granulocyte macrophage (CFU-GM) numbers were greatly diminished. Administration of PSBS reconstituted myelopoiesis, with the number of CFU-GM increasing about 1.8-fold in 5-FU-treated mice, when compared with the 5-FU alone group. None of the PSBS-treated mice died, nor did their body weights change significantly during the experimental period (Liao et al., 2005).

(4-Methoxyphenyl)(3,4,5-trimethoxyphenyl)methanone (PHT) - PHT is a phenstatin analog. PHT is a known tubulin inhibitor that has potent cytotoxic activity (Magalhães et al., 2011a, 2011b). Using S-180-bearing mice, Magalhães et al. (2011a) observed a reduction in tumor weight in PHT-treated animals as well as for the PHT plus 5-FU-treated animals. The authors determined hematological parameters (platelet count and total and differential leukocyte counts) of these animals. Unlike several chemotherapeutics, PHT did not reduce the number of hematopoietic cells. However, treatment with PHT combined with 5-FU positively influenced the increase in total leukocytes (Magalhães, 2011a).

Sulfated Polysaccharide from the Red Seaweed Champia feldmannii (Diaz-Pifferer) - Sulfated-polysaccharides are complex macromolecular constituents of the extracellular matrix of marine algae. From *C. feldmannii*, a sulfated polysaccharide (Cf-PLS) has been isolated. This molecule has demonstrated a potent edematogenic activity associated with an increased vascular permeability and stimulation of neutrophil migration (Assreuy et al., 2008). Lins et al. (2009), using Sarcoma 180-bearing mice, demonstrated that Cf-PLS (10 and 25 mg/kg) inhibited S-180 tumor growth in mice. When the tumor-bearing animals were treated simultaneously with both the sulfated polysaccharide (10 mg/kg) and the chemotherapeutic agent, 5-FU (10 mg/kg), the tumor inhibition rate increased significantly. The authors also found an increase in the relative spleen weight, the presence of hyperplasia of lymphoid follicles with nests of megakaryocyte-like cells in the spleen, and a prevention of the leukopenia induced by 5-FU in treated animals, probably due to immunological stimulation.

Latex of Calotropis procera - Latex of *Calotropis procera* has been described as a relevant source of pharmacologically active proteins, including proteins with anticancer activity (Oliveira et al., 2010). Although rubber predominates, the latex of *C. procera* is a rich source of proteins (LP) (Freitas et al., 2007). Oliveira et al. (2010) found that the LP significantly reduced *in vivo* tumor growth in a dose-dependent manner (both intraperitoneal and oral routes of administration) in S-180-bearing animals. They also observed that the life span of the animals that received LP was increased. When the animals were treated with LP (2 mg/kg) plus 5-FU (10 mg/kg) via intraperitoneal route or LP (10 mg/kg) plus 5-FU (10 mg/kg) via oral route, the leukopenia induced by 5-FU was also diminished.

Piplartine - Piplartine is a biologically active component from the *Piper* species (Piperaceae), which have high economical and medicinal importance. Piplartine inhibited sarcoma 180 tumor growth in mice after the administration of 7 doses of 50 or 100 mg/kg, showing an *in vivo* antitumor effect (Bezerra et al., 2006). Besides this, when the tumor-bearing animals were treated with piplartine plus 5-FU, the tumor inhibition rate increased additively (Bezerra et al., 2008a). Additionally, leukocytopenia was observed with 5-FU treatment alone, which was prevented by the association with piplartine, indicating a protective effect of piplartine against delayed hematopoietic depression induced by 5-FU. The combination of piplartine and 5-FU did not induce substantial changes in biochemical, hematological and histopathological parameters. It is possible that this combination augments the antitumor activity without augmenting side effects, and, moreover, it could even attenuate 5-FU toxicity (Bezerra et al., 2008a).

Anthocyanin-rich extract from bilberry (Vaccinium myrtillus L.) - Anthocyanins are a group of plant pigments that are extensively distributed in nature (Hou et al., 2012). Choi et al. (2007) tested anthocyanin-rich extract from bilberry (AREB) using 5-FU-induced myelotoxicity from a single dose (200 mg/kg, i.p.) in a treatment over 10 days. The oral administration of AREB resulted in considerable improvement of the hematological parameters such as red blood cells, hemoglobin, hematocrit, platelets, white blood cells, lymphocytes, neutrophils, and monocytes that were all reduced by 5-FU. The AREB treatment also increased the number of splenic cells as well as the number of bone marrow nucleated cells, compared with the 5-FU alone group, in a dose-dependent manner (Choi et al., 2007).

CF101 - CF101 is an A_3 adenosine receptor (A_3AR) agonist. Ohana et al. (2003) tested the effect of CF101 on the growth of human HCT-116 and murine CT-26 colon carcinoma cells. Mice treated with 5-FU exhibited a decline in the number of peripheral blood leukocytes and absolute neutrophil counts. Administration of CF101 following chemotherapy increased the number of white blood cells and restored the percentage of neutrophils (Ohana et al., 2003).

Others - Other drugs have also shown a preventive effect on 5-FU-induced myelotoxicity, such as: *Scutellaria baicalensis* Georgii extract (Razina et al., 1987); *Potassium oxonate* (Kouchi et al., 2002); Rosiglitazone (Djazayeri et al., 2005); and an acidic glycoprotein prepared from a culture of *Chlorella vulgaris* (Konichi, 1996).

CONCLUSION

The ability to predict myelosuppression/immunosuppression after 5-FU administration is important in making treatment choices for cancer patients; eventually, cytotoxic regimens will be adapted to the expected tolerance of the patient. Herein, the clinical immunological effects of 5-FU, as well as experimental models used to assess and identify new compounds to treat 5-FU-induced immunotoxicity, were summarized. Different compounds have been described in literature as agents able to prevent/reduce the 5-FU-induced immunotoxicity, including chitosans and polysaccharides. In the future, further details of the mechanism and compositional analysis of theses extracts/compounds should be studied experimentally and through controlled clinical evaluations.

REFERENCES

Amstutz, U; Froehlich, TK; Largiadèr, CR. Dihydropyrimidine dehydrogenase gene as a major predictor of severe 5-fluorouracil toxicity. *Pharmacogenomics*, 2011, 12, 1321-36.

Aranda, E; Cervantes, A; Carrato, A; Fernandez-Martos, C; Anton-Torres, A; Massuti T; Barneto, I; García-Conde, J; Barón, JM; Díaz-Rubio, E and Spanish Cooperative Group For Gastrointestinal Tumor Therapy. Outpatient weekly high-dose continuous infusion 5-fluorouracil plus oral leucovorin in advanced colorectal cancer. A phase II trial. Spanish Cooperative Group for Gastrointestinal Tumor Therapy (TTD). *Annals of Oncology*, 1996, 7, 581–585.

Aranda, E; Cervantes, A; Carrato, A; Fernández-Martos, C; Antón-Torres, A; Massutí, T; Barneto, I; García-Conde, J; Barón, JM; Díaz-Rubio, E. A phase II trial of weekly high dose continuous infusion 5-fluorouracil plus oral leucovorin in patients with advanced colorectal cancer. The Spanish Cooperative Group for Gastrointestinal Tumor Therapy (TTD). *Cancer*, 1995, 76, 559-563.

Aranda, E; Diaz-Rubio, E; Cervantes, A; Anton-Torres, A; Carrato, A; Massuti, T; Tabernero, JM; Sastre, J; Trés, A; Aparicio, J; López-Vega, JM; Barneto, I; García-Conde, J. and on behalf of the Spanish Cooperative Group for Gastrointestinal Tumor Therapy (TTD). Randomized trial comparing monthly low-dose leucovorin and fluorouracil bolus with weekly high-dose 48-h continuous infusion fluorouracil for advanced colorectal cancer: a Spanish Cooperative Group for Gastrointestinal Tumor Therapy (TTD) study. *Annals of Oncology*, 1998, 727–731.

Ardalan, B; Chua, L; Tian, EM; Reddy, R; Sridhar, K; Benedetto, P; Richman, S; Legaspi, A; Waldman, S; Morrell. A phase II study of weekly 24-h infusion with high-dose fluorouracil with leucovorin in colorectal carcinoma. *Journal of Clinical Oncology*, 1991, 9, 625-630.

Asanuma, F; Miyata, H; Iwaki, Y; Kimura, M; Matsumoto, K. Evaluation of short-term myelotoxicity study in dietary reduced rats. *Journal* of Toxicologic Pathology, 2010, 23, 31–37.

Assef, MLM.; Carneiro-Leão, AM; Moretão, MP; Azambuja, AP; Lacomini, M; Buchi, DF. Histological and immunohistochemical evaluation of Sarcoma 180 in mice after treatment with an α-d-glucan from the lichen *Ramalina celastri*. *Brazilian Journal of Morphological Science*, 2002, 19, 49-54.

Assreuy, MAS; Gomes, DM; Silva, MSJ; Torres, VM; Siqueira, RCL; Pires, AF; Criddle, DN; Alencar, NMN; Cavada, BS; Sampaio, AH;, Farias, WR. Biological effects of a sulphated polysaccharide isolated from the marine red algae *Champia feldmannii*. *Biological and Pharmaceutical Bulletin*, 2008, 31, 691-695.

Beerblock, K; Rinaldi, Y; Andre, T; Louvet, C; Raymond, E; Tournigand, C; Carola, E; Favre, R; de Gramont, A; Krulik M. Bimonthly high dose leucovorin and 5-fluorouracil 48-h continuous infusion in patients with advanced colorectal carcinoma. Groupe d'Etude et de Recherche sur les Cancers de l'Ovaire et Digestifs (GERCOD). *Cancer*, 1997, 79, 1100-1105.

Bezerra, DP; Castro, FO; Alves, AP; Pessoa, C; Moraes, MO; Silveira, ER; Lima, MA; Elmiro, FJ; Alencar, NM; Mesquita, RO; Lima, MW; Costa-Lotufo, LV. *In vitro* and *in vivo* antitumor effect of 5-FU combined with piplartine and piperine. *Journal of Applied Toxicology,* 2008a, 28, 156-163.

Bezerra, DP; Castro, FO; Alves, APNN; Pessoa, C; Moraes, MO; Silveira, ER; Lima, MAS; Elmiro, FJM; Costa-Lotufo, LV. *In vivo* growth-inhibition of Sarcoma 180 by piplartine and piperine, two alkaloid amides from *Piper*. *Brazilian Journal of Medical and Biological Research,* 2006, 39, 801-807.

Bezerra, DP; Pessoa, C; Moraes, MO; Alencar, NM; Mesquita, RO; Lima, MW; Alves, AP; Pessoa, OD; Chaves, JH; Silveira, ER; Costa-Lotufo, LV. *In vivo* growth inhibition of sarcoma 180 by piperlonguminine, an alkaloid amide from the *Piper* species. *Journal of Applied Toxicology,* 2008b, 28, 599-607.

Buroker, TR; O'Connell, MJ; Wieand, HS; Krook, JE; Gerstner, JB; Mailliard, JA; Schaefer, PL; Levitt, R; Kardinal, CG; Gesme, DH Jr. Randomized comparison of two schedules of fluorouracil and leucovorin in the treatment of advanced colorectal cancer. *Journal of Clinical Oncology,* 1994, 12, 14-20.

Chen, X; Zhang, L; Cheung, PC. Immunopotentiation and anti-tumor activity of carboxymethylated-sulfated β-(1-3)-d-glucan from *Poria cocos. International Immunopharmacology*, 2010, 10, 398-405.

Choi, CW; Sung, HJ; Park, KH; Yoon, SY; Kim, SJ; Oh, SC; Seo, JH; Kim, BS; Shin, SW; Kim, YH; Kim JS. Early lymphopenia as a risk factor for chemotherapy-induced febrile neutropenia. *American Journal of Hematology,* 2003, 73, 263-266.

Choi, EH; Oka, HE; Yoon, Y; Magnuson, BA; Kim, MK; Chuna, HS. Protective effect of anthocyanin-rich extract from bilberry (*Vaccinium myrtillus* L.) against myelotoxicity induced by 5-fluorouracil. *BioFactors*, 2007, 29, 55-65.

Ciccolini, J; Gross, E; Dahan, L; Lacarelle, B; Mercier, C. Routine dihydropyrimidine dehydrogenase testing for anticipating 5-fluorouracil-related severe toxicities: hype or hope? *Clinical Colorectal Cancer*, 2010, 9, 224-228.

Dale, DC. Colony-stimulating factors for the management of neutropaenia in cancer patients. *Drugs*, 2002, 62, 1-15.

Dasha, M; Chiellini, F; Ottenbriteb, RM; Chiellini, E. Chitosan: A versatile semi-synthetic polymer in biomedical applications. *Progress in Polymer Science*, 2011, 36, 981-1014.

De Gramont, A; Bosset, JF; Milan, C; Rougier, P; Bouche, O; Etienne, PL; Morvan, F; Louvet, C; Guillot, T; François, E; Bedenne, L. Randomized trial comparing monthly low-dose leucovorin and fluorouracil bolus with bimonthly high-dose leucovorin and fluorouracil bolus plus continuous infusion for advanced colorectal cancer: a French intergroup study. *Journal of Clinical Oncology*, 1997, 15, 808-815.

De Gramont, A; Louvet, C; Andre, T; Tournigand, C; Krulik, M. A review of GERCOD trials of bimonthly leucovorin plus 5-fluorouracil 48-h continuous infusion in advanced colorectal cancer: evolution of a regimen. Groupe d'Etude et de Recherche sur les Cancers de l'Ovaire et Digestifs (GERCOD). *European Journal of Cancer*, 1998, 34, 619-626.

Diaz-Rubio, E; Aranda, E; Martin, M; Gonzalez-Mancha, R; Gonzalez-Larriba, J; Barneto, I. Weekly high-dose infusion of 5-fluorouracil in advanced colorectal cancer. *European Journal of Cancer,* 1990, 26, 727-729.

Djazayeri, K; Szilvássy, Z; Peitl, B; Németh, J; Nagy, L; Kiss, A; Szabó, B; Benkő, I. Accelerated recovery of 5-fluorouracil-damaged bone marrow after rosiglitazone treatment. *European Journal of Pharmacology*, 2005, 522, 122-129.

Flemming, WH; Weissman, IL. Haematopoietic stem cells. In: Abeloff M.D., Armitage J.O., Lichter A.S.; Neiderhuber J.E., Eds Clinical Oncology. Churchill Livingstone. 1995, 127-133.

Freitas, CD; Oliveira, JS; Miranda, MR; Macedo, NM; Sales, MP; Villas-boas, LA; Ramos, MV. Enzymatic activities and protein profile of latex from Calotropis procera. *Plant Physiology and Biochemistry,* 2007, 45, 781-789.

Gladysheva, IP; Moroz, NA; Karmakova, TA; Nemtsova, ER; Yakubovskaya, RI; Larionova, NI. Immunoconjugates of soybean Bowman-Birk protease inhibitor as targeted antitumor polymeric agents. *Journal of Drug Targeting*, 2001, 9, 303-316.

Gonzaga, MLC; Bezerra, DP; Alves, APNN; Alencar, NMN; Mesquita, RO; Lima, MW; Soares, SA; Pessoa, C; Moraes, MO; Costa-Lotufo, LV. *In vivo* growth-inhibition of Sarcoma 180 by an α-(1-4)-glucanβ-(1-6)-glucan-protein complex polysaccharide obtained from Agaricus blazei Murill. *Journal of Natural Medicines*, 2009, 63, 32-40.

Ho, YF; Lu, WC; Chen, RR; Cheng, AL; Yeh, KH. Phase I, pharmacokinetic, and bone marrow drug-level studies of tri-monthly 48-h infusion of high-dose 5-fluorouracil and leucovorin in patients with metastatic colorectal cancers. *Anticancer Drugs*, 2011, 22, 290-298.

Hou, Z; Qin, P; Zhang, Y; Cui, S; Ren, G. Identification of anthocyanins isolated from black rice (*Oryza sativa* L.) and the degradation kinetics. *Food Research International*, 2012, *in press*.

Katzung, GB. Basic and Clinical Pharmacology, 9th edition, 2003, USA: McGraw-Hill Medical.

Kimura, Y. Prevention of cancer chemotherapy drug-induced adverse reaction, antitumor and antimetastatic activities by natural products. *Studies in Natural Products Chemistry*, 2003, 28, 559-589.

Kimura, Y.; Okuda, H. Prevention by chitosan of myelotoxicity, gastrointestinal toxicity and immunocompetent organic toxicity induced by 5-fluorouracil without loss of antitumor activity in mice. *Japanese Journal of Cancer Research,* 1999a, 90, 765-774.

Kimura, Y; Okuda, H. Prevention by carp extract of myelotoxicity and gastrointestinal toxicity induced by 5-fluorouracil without loss of antitumor activity in mice. *Journal of Ethnopharmacology*, 1999b, 68, 39-45.

Kobayashi, K; Abe, Y; Kuriyama, K. Whole blood TNF-α production as a sensitive measure for immunotoxicity of anticancer drugs. *Journal of Toxicological Sciences*, 2006, 31, 71-74.

Konishi, F; Mitsuyama, M; Okuda, M; Tanaka, K; Hasegawa, T; Nomoto, K. Protective effect of an acidic glycoprotein obtained from culture of *Chlorella vulgaris* against myelosuppression by 5-fluorouracil. *Cancer Immunology Immunotherapy*, 1996, 42, 268-274.

Kouchi, Y; Maeda, Y; Ohuchida, A; Nomura, N. Potassium oxonate modulation of 5-fluorouracil-induced myelotoxicity in murine and human colony forming assays of hematopoietic precursor cells. *Toxicology Letters*, 2002, 135, 11-18.

Lee, IP; Kang, BH; Roh, JK; Kim, JR. Lack of carcinogenicity of lyophilized *Agaricus blazei* Murill in a F344 rat two year bioassay. *Food and Chemical Toxicology*, 2008, 46, 87-95.

Lee, JH; Cho, KM. Changes occurring in compositional components of black soybeans maintained at room temperature for different storage periods. *Food Chemistry*, 2012, 131, 161-169.

Liao, HF; Chen, TYJ; Yang, YC. A novel polysaccharide of black soybean promotes myelopoiesis and reconstitutes bone marrow after 5-flurouracil- and irradiation-induced myelosuppression. *Life Sciences*, 2005, 77, 400–413.

Lins, KO; Bezerra, DP; Alves, AP; Alencar, NM; Lima, MW; Torres, VM; Farias, WR; Pessoa, C; Moraes, MO; Costa-Lotufo, LV. Antitumor properties of a sulfated polysaccharide from the red seaweed *Champia feldmannii* (Diaz-Pifferer). *Journal of Applied Toxicology*, 2009, 29, 20-26.

Longley, DB; Harkin, DP; Johnston, PG. 5-fluorouracil: mechanisms of action and clinical strategies. *Nature Reviews Cancer*, 2003, 3, 330-308.

Lorenza, M; Slaughtera, HS; Wescotta, DM; Cartera, SI; Schnydera, B; Dinchuka, JE; Car, BD. Cyclooxygenase-2 is essential for normal recovery from 5-fluorouracil–induced myelotoxicity in mice. *Experimental Hematology*, 2010, 27, 1494-1502.

Macdonald, JS. Toxicity of 5-fluorouracil. *Oncology*, 1999, 13, 33-34.

Magalhães, HIF; Bezerra, DP; Cavalcanti, BC; Wilke, DV; Rotta, R; De Lima, DP; Beatriz, A; Alves, APNN; Bitencourt, FS; Figueiredo, IST; Alencar, NMN; Costa-Lotufo, LV; Moraes, MO; Pessoa, C. *In vitro* and *in vivo* antitumor effects of (4-methoxyphenyl)(3,4,5-trimethoxyphenyl)methanone. *Cancer Chemotherapy and Pharmacology*, 2011a, 68, 45-52.

Magalhães, HIF; Cavalcanti, BC; Bezerra, DP; Wilke, DV; Paiva, JCG; Rotta, R; De Lima, DP; Beatriz, A; Burbano, RR; Costa-Lotufo, LV; Moraes, MO; Pessoa, C. Assessment of genotoxic effects of (4-methoxyphenyl)(3,4,5-trimethoxyphenyl)methanone in human lymphocytes. *Toxicology In Vitro*, 2011b, 25, 2048-2053.

Malet-Martino, M; Martino, R. Clinical studies of three oral prodrugs of 5-fluorouracil (capecitabine, UFT, S-1): a review. *Oncologist*, 2002, 7, 288-323.

Minemoto, Y; Fang, X; Hakamata, K; Watanabe, Y; Adachi, S; Kometani, T; Matsuno, R. Oxidation of linoleic acid encapsulated with soluble soybean polysaccharide by spray-drying. *Bioscience, Biotechnology and Biochemistry*, 2002, 66, 1829-1834.

Mitchell, JA; Gillam, EM; Stanley, LA; Sim, E. Immunotoxic side-effects of drug therapy. *Drug Safety*, 1990, 5, 168-178.

Mosmann, TR; Sad, S. The expanding universe of T-cell subsets: Th1, Th2 and more. *Immunology Today*, 1996, 17, 138-145.

Niu, G; Tan, J; Turner, JG; Brabham, JG; Burdelya, LG; Crucian, BE; Wall-Apelt, H; Zhao, RJ; Yu, H. Bing de ling, a Chinese herbal formula, stimulates multifaceted immunologic responses in mice. *DNA and Cell Biology*, 2000, 19, 515-520.

Numazawa, S; Sugihara, K; Miyake, S; Tomiyama. H; Hida, A; Hatsuno, M; Yamamoto, M; Yoshida T. Possible involvement of oxidative stress in 5-fluorouracil-mediated myelosuppression in mice. *Basic and Clinical Pharmacology and Toxicology*, 2011, 108, 40-45.

Ogawa, M. Differentiation and proliferation of haematopoietic stem cells. Blood, 1993, 81, 2844-2853.

Ohana, O; Bar-Yehuda, S; Arich, A; Mad, L; Dreznick, Z; Rath-Wolfson, L; Silberman, D; Slosman, G; Fishman, P. Inhibition of primary colon carcinoma growth and liver metastasis by the A3 adenosine receptor agonist CF101. *British Journal of Cancer*, 2003, 89, 1552–1558.

Ohta, Y; Sueki, K; Kitta, K; Takemoto, K.; Ishitsuka, H; Yagi, Y. Comparative studies on the immunosuppressive effect among 5'-deoxy 5-fluorouridine, ftorafur, and 5-fluorouracil. *Gann*, 1980, 71, 190-196.

Oliveira, JS; Costa-Lotufo, LV; Bezerra, DP; Alencar, NMN; Marinho-Filho, JDB; Figueiredo, IST; Moraes, MO; Pessoa, C; Alves, ANN; Ramos, M. *In vivo* growth inhibition of sarcoma 180 by latex proteins from *Calotropis procera*. *Naunyn-Schmiedeberg's Archives of Pharmacology*, 2010, 382, 139-149.

Ozer, H; Armitage, JO; Bennett, CL; Crawford, J; Demetri, GD; Pizzo, PA; Schiffer, CA; Smith, TJ; Somlo, G; Wade, JC; Wade, JL; Winn, RJ; Wozniak, AJ; Somerfield, MR. American Society of Clinical Oncology. Update of recommendations for the use of haematopoietic colonystimulating factors: Evidence-based, clinical practice guidelines. *Journal of Clinical Oncology,* 2000, 18, 3558-3585.

Pettengell, R; Gurney, H; Radford, JA; Deakin, DP; James, R; Wilkinson, PM; Kane, K; Bentley, J; Crowther, D. Granulocyte colony-stimulating factor to prevent dose-limiting neutropenia in non-Hodgkin's lymphoma: a randomized controlled trial. *Blood*, 1992, 80, 1430-1436.

Poon, MA; O'Connell, MJ; Wieand, HS; Krook, JE; Gerstner, JB; Tschetter, LK; Levitt, R; Kardinal, CG; Mailliard, JA. Biochemical modulation of fluorouracil with leucovorin: confirmatory evidence of improved therapeutic efficacy in advanced colorectal cancer. *Journal of Clinical Oncology,* 1991, 9, 1967-1972.

Rairakhwada, D; Pal, AK; Bhathena, ZP; Sahu, NP; Jha, A; Mukherjee, SJ. Dietary microbial levan enhances cellular non-specific immunity and survival of common carp (Cyprinus carpio) juveniles. *Fish and Shellfish Immunology*, 2007, 22, 477-486.

Razina, TG; Udintsev, SN; Prishchep, TP; Iaremenko, KV. Enhancement of the selectivity of the action of the cytostatics cyclophosphane and 5-fluorouracil by using an extract of the Baikal skullcap in an experiment. *Vopr Onkol.*, 1987, 33, 80-84.

Shah, A; MacDonald, W; Goldie, J; Gudauskas, G; Brisebois, B. 5-FU infusion in advanced colorectal cancer: a comparison of three dose schedules. *Cancer Treatment Reports*, 1985, 69, 739-742.

Shibata, Y; Fujita, S; Takahashi, H; Yamaguchi, A; Koji, T. Assessment of decalcifying protocols for detection of specific RNA by non-radioactive in situ hybridization in calcified tissues. *Histochemistry and Cell Biology*, 2000, 113, 153-159.

Spicer, DV; Ardalan, B; Daniels, JR; Silberman, H; Johnson, K. Reevaluation of the maximum tolerated dose of continuous venous infusion of 5-fluorouracil with pharmacokinetics. *Cancer Research*, 1988, 48, 459-461.

Suzuki, K; Koike, H; Matsui, H; Ono, Y; Hasumi, M; Nakazato, H; Okugi, H; Sekine, Y; Oki, K; Ito, K; Yamamoto, T; Fukabori, Y; Kurokawa, K; Yamanaka, H. Genistein, a soy isoflavone, induces glutathione peroxidase in the human prostate cancer cell lines LNCaP and PC-3. *International Journal of Cancer*, 2002, 99, 846-852.

Tavassoli, M. Embryonic and total haematopoiesis. *Blood*, 1991, 17, 269-281.

Timeus, F; Crescenzio, N; Saracco, P; Doria, A; Fazio, L; Albiani, R; Cordero, Di; Montezemolo, L; Perugini, L; Incarbone, E. Recovery of cord blood hematopoietic progenitors after successive freezing and thawing procedures. *Haematologica*, 2003, 88, 74-79.

Wang, SY; Hsu, ML; Su, CY; Lin, CK; Hu, CP; Chang, C. *In vivo* stimulation of myelopoiesis in cyclophosphamide-treated mice by purified human GM-CSF. *Chinese Medical Journal*, 1991, 48, 171-176.

Wang, SY; Wang, RC; Chen, LY; Lieu, CW; Su, SN; Yung, CH; Ho, CK. Purification and characterization of human macrophage-derived granulomonopoietic enhancing factor (GM-EF). *Experimental Hematology*, 1992, 20, 552-557.

Xu, Q; Brabham, JG; Zhang, S; Munster, P; Fields, K; Zhao, R-J; Yu, H. Chinese herbal formula, Bing de Ling, enhances antitumor effects and ameliorates weight loss induced by 5-fluorouracil in the mouse CT26 tumor model. *DNA and Cell Biology*, 2005, 24, 470-475.

Yeh, KH; Cheng, AL. An alternative method to overcome central venous portable external infusion pump blockage in patients receiving weekly 24-h high-dose fluorouracil and leucovorin. *Journal of Clinical Oncology*, 1994, 12, 875-876.

Yeh, KH; Cheng, AL; Lin, MT; Hong, RL; Hsu, CH; Lin, JF; Chang, KJ; Lee, PH; Chen, YC. A phase II study of weekly 24-h infusion of high-dose 5-fluorouracil and leucovorin (HDFL) in the treatment of recurrent or metastatic colorectal cancers. *Anticancer Research*, 1997, 17, 3867-3871.

Yeh, KH; Yeh, SH; Chang, YS; Cheng, AL. Minimal toxicity to myeloid progenitor cells of weekly 24-h infusion of high-dose 5-fluorouracil: direct evidence from colony-forming unit granulocyte and monocyte (CFU-GM) clonogenic assay. *Pharmacology and Toxicology*, 2000a, 86, 122-124.

Yeh, KH; Yeh, SH; Hsu, CH; Wang, TM; Ma, IF; Cheng, AL. Prolonged and enhanced suppression of thymidylate synthase by weekly 24-h infusion of high-dose 5-fluorouracil. *British Journal of Cancer*, 2000b, 83, 1510-1515.

Young, HA; Hardy, KJ. Role of interferon-gamma in immune cell regulation. *Journal of Leukocyte Biology,* 1995, 58, 373-381.

Zheng, Y; Zhou, F; Wu, X; Wen, X; Li, Y; Yan, B; Zhang, J; Hao, G; Ye, W; Wang, G. 23-hydroxybetulinic acid from *Pulsatilla chinensis* (Bunge) Regel synergizes the antitumor activities of doxorubicin *in vitro* and *in vivo*. *Journal of Ethnopharmacology*, 2010, 128, 615-622.

In: Fluorouracil
Editors: A. Longinho and S. Dobreiro

ISBN: 978-1-62081-970-8
© 2012 Nova Science Publishers, Inc.

Chapter IV

FLUOROURACIL (5FU) – USING AND SIDE EFFECTS

Claudio Sergio Batista[1,2,3,4,5,6], *Telma Lima Martins*[1,7,8,9] *and Fernanda Carvalhido Antonio Batista*[10]

[1]Faculty of Medicine of Petropolis, Rio de Janeiro, Brazil
[2]Program of Post-Graduation in Internal and Therapeutical Medicine,
Federal University of São Paulo/São Paulo School of Medicine,
São Paulo, Brazil
[3]Effectiveness in Evidence-Based Medicine,
Federal University of São Paulo/São Paulo School of Medicine,
São Paulo, Brazil
[4]Gynecology and Obstetrics for the Brazilian Federation of the Society of
Gynecology and Obstetrics/Brazilian Medical Association
(FEBRASGO/AMB), Brazil
[5]Pontifical University Catholic of Rio de Janeiro, Brazil
[6]Corpo de Bombeiros Militar do Estado do Rio de Janeiro, Brazil
[7]Federal University of São Paulo/São Paulo School of Medicine,
São Paulo, Brazil
[8]Cardiology, (SBC/AMB), Brazil
[9]Cardiology, School of Post-Graduate of Rio de Janeiro, Brazil
[10]School of Medicine of Fundação Tecnico Educacional Souza Marques,
Rio de Janeiro, Brazil

ABSTRACT

Fluorouracil is a fluorinated pyrimidine anti-metabolite that functions as an anti-neoplastic agent by blocking DNA and RNA synthesis and stopping the growth of cancer cells. Once administered, the drug is concentrated especially on neoplastic tissue. Fluorouracil is used to treat several types of cancer including colon, rectum and head and neck cancers. It is also used for other types of cancer, and the skin cream is used for other conditions as well as skin neoplasms and precancerous lesions, such as actinic keratosis, and also for non-malignant lesions as genital warts. Commonly, Fluorouracil can cause side effects such as low platelet and white blood cell count, darkening of skin and nail beds, nausea and vomiting, poor appetite, sores in mouth, lips, or throat, hair loss or thinning, diarrhea, brittle nails, increased sensitivity to sun, dry, flaky and cracking skin. Less commonly, it can raise darkening and hardening of veins used for giving the drug, headache, weakness, muscle aches, and rarely can provoke trouble walking, trouble forming words, and poor coordination, irritated eyes, increased tears, watering eyes, blurred vision, heart problems, confusion, tingling, numbness, or swelling in the hands and feet, and severe allergic reaction. Despite those side effects, Fluorouracil is a safe drug for the treatment of cancers cited above.

FLUOROURACIL (5FU) – USAGE AND SIDE EFFECTS

1. Introduction

Chemotherapy for the treatment of cancer was introduced into the clinic more than fifty years ago. Although this form of therapy has been successful for the treatment of some tumors such as testicular cancer and certain leukemias, its success for the treatment of common epithelial tumors of the breast, colon, and lung has been less than spectacular. Ideally, chemotherapeutic drugs should specifically target and should decrease tumor burden by inducing cyto and/or cytostatic effects with minimal "collateral damage" to normal cells. In reality, the effectiveness has suffered from a range of confounding factors including systemic toxicity due to a lack of specificity, rapid drug metabolism, and both intrinsic and acquired drug resistance. The problem of multidrug resistance has been the least understood, and most unpredictable factor affecting chemotherapy. Given the adaptability of tumor cells, it seems likely that drug resistance will continue to be an important clinical problem, even in the age of targeted therapeutics and tailored treatment regimes. (Johnstone, et al., 2002)

Since most cancer drugs were identified using empirical screens, the molecular events responsible for their anti-tumor effect were poorly understood. Over the last decade, our understanding of cellular damage responses and physiological cell death mechanisms has improved, leading, in turn, to new insights into drug-induced cell. Drugs of differing structure and specificity induce the characteristic morphological changes associated with apoptosis, and it is now believed that apoptosis contributes to the cytotoxic action of most chemotherapeutic drugs (Lowe et al, 2000).

Collectively, these observations indicate that cells can interpret a drug-induced insult in the same way that a physiological insult, such as hypoxia or growth factor deprivation, is interpreted. Since the efficiency of apoptosis depends on an elaborate molecular network, the killing of tumor cells by anti-cancer agents may be remarkably indirect (Johnstone et al., 2002).

A variation on the theme of rational drug design is the idea of individualized therapy whereby the "cure circumvents the cause." Theoretically, a more targeted approach to chemotherapy might involve genotyping individual tumors for their drug resistance profiles, and then employing agents known to work effectively despite the identified anti-apoptotic lesions. The potential of this approach is illustrated by a study demonstrating that tumor cells with elevated levels of c-*myc* and wild-type p53 are selectively sensitive to 5-FU (Arango et al., 2001).

5-fluorouracil (FU) is one of the oldest anti-cancer drugs, and its use in cancer chemotherapy continues to increase. It is a pro-drug that requires intracellular activation to exert its effects (Milano and Chamorey, 2002).

5-Fluorouracil is an anti-metabolite fluoropyrimidine analog of the nucleoside pyrimidine with anti-neoplastic activity. Fluorouracil and its metabolites possess a number of different mechanisms of action. In vivo, fluoruracil is converted to the active metabolite 5-fluoroxyuridine monophosphate (F-UMP); replacing uracil, F-UMP incorporates into RNA and inhibits RNA processing, thereby inhibiting cell growth. Another active metabolite, 5-5-fluoro-2'-deoxyuridine-5'-O-monophosphate (F-dUMP), inhibits thymidylate synthase, resulting in the depletion of thymidine triphosphate (TTP), one of the four nucleotide triphosphates used in the in vivo synthesis of DNA. Other fluorouracil metabolites incorporate into both RNA and DNA; incorporation into RNA results in major effects on both RNA processing and functions (NCI, 2012).

As it is a part of a group of chemotherapy drugs known as the anti-metabolites, 5-FU is similar to normal body molecules but they have a slightly different structure. These differences mean that anti-metabolites stop cells working properly. They stop cells making and repairing DNA. Cancer cells need to make and repair DNA in order to grow and multiply. Anti-metabolites also stop normal cells working properly and cause side effects.

2. Usage

Chemotherapy is usually given as a course of several sessions or cycles of treatment over a few months. The length of your treatment and the number of cycles depends on the type of cancer for which you are being treated. 5-FU may be given by intravenously, orally or applied directly to the skin as a cream or ointment.

5-Fluorouracil is also known as FU or 5-FU and is one of the most commonly used drugs to treat cancer, and it has been used and considered a mainstay for treating various solid tumors in adults including breast cancer, head and neck cancers, anal cancer, stomach cancer, colon cancer and some skin cancers besides to be used for treating others conditions such as some benign skin disease as sun keratosis, actinic keratosis and genital warts (Cordier et al., 2011)

Although the Food and Drug Administration (FDA) has not approved the use of 5-FU for genital warts, it is being used as 5% cream by physicians as a result of uncontrolled clinical trials. As a topical application, this anti-metabolite drug is more commonly used to treat a variety of skin neoplasms and precancerous lesions, such as actinic keratosis. It has been used by clinicians for treating urethral condylomata for 20 years. It can also be used on more routine anogenital condylomata, whether apparent or sub-clinical, with good effect (Dyment 1996).

Frequently, 5-FU has been evaluated as a 5% topical cream or solution and as an adjunct to laser therapy for severe vulvar diseases. An injectable 3% preparation in a collagen gel with epinephrine for vasoconstriction has also been utilized (Dyment 1996, Batista 2010).

5-FU also can be used in ophthalmic surgery, specifically trabeculectomy, the surgery to aim to diminish intraocular pressure in patients with glaucoma. It also may used in pterygium surgery for preventing relapse (Schellini et al., 2000; Shiratori et al., 2003; Valezi et al., 2009)

As for non-malignant conditions, the doses are often lower than for cancer treatment and the side effects may be reduced, but they may always be present as for any drug utilization.

5-FU has been used alone or in addition with other drugs such as leucovorin, irinotecan, oxaliplatin, leucovorin with oxaliplatin, leucovorin and irinotecan combination therapy, doxorubicin, cyclophosphamide, paclitaxel depending of types of cancer, and the schemes are varied in dose, time and type of infusion (continuous or in bolus) (Meta-analysis Group in Cancer, 1998; Wilkes, 2005)

Some schemes are used according to the types of cancer as well as: CAF (Ciclofosmamida, Adriamicin(Doxorubicin), Fluorouracil) for breast cancer, CMF (Ciclofosfamida, Metrotexate, Fluorouracil) for breast cancer, FEC (Fluorouracil, Epirubicin, Ciclofosfamifda) for breast cancer, ECF (Epirubicin, Cisplatina, Fluorouracil) for stomach and esofagus cancer, FOLFOX (Fluorouracil, Leucovorin (Folinic acid), Oxaliplatin) for colorectal cancer, 5-FU/Leucovorin - 6 months, (NCCTG), 5-FU/Leucovorin – high dose/week/ 6 months (NSABP), 5-FU/Levamisole/ year as adjuvant to colorectal cancer (O'Connell et al., 1997; Wolmark; 1999; Moertel, 1994)

5-FU dose by endovenous pathway ranges from 6 mg/Kg/day to 12 mg/Kg/day and must not exceed 800 mg/m^2/day, by intra-arterial via the dose ranges from 10 to 800 mg/m^2/day, and by oral via ranges from 20/mg/Kg/day to 15 mg/kg/week.

5-FU is available in Brazil as capsula of 250 mg, as skin cream and as injectable solution ranging of 10 mg/mL, 25mg/mL, to 50 mg/mL. In the USA and Europe it is available as capsula of 250 mg, as cream of 10 mg/g or 50 mg/g, as topical solution of 10 mg/mL, 20 mg/mL or 50 mg/mL, and as injectable solution of 25 mg/mL, 50 mg/mL.

Some studies have shown that long-term exposure of ailing tissues to moderate drug concentrations is more favorable than regular administration of higher concentration of the drug, and its results indicate the potential of 5-FU-loaded poly-lactic-*co*-glycolic acid (PLGA) nanoparticles with dependence on carrier combination as controlled release formulation to multiply the therapeutic effect of *cancer* chemotherapy (Nair, 2011)

3. Side Effects

Concerning side effects, it has observed that chemotherapy is not free as well as any drug and medicine, and for each person, chemotherapy reaction is different, and in some people we can see very few side effects, while others may experience more. The side effects are also different if using only a drug or using drugs in association.

The often debilitating side effects of chemotherapy are a major clinical problem. Although chemotherapeutic drugs would ideally specifically target only tumor cells, hemopoietic and intestinal epithelial cells, and hair matrix keratinocytes are often susceptible to the toxic effects of these agents (Komarova and Gudkov, 2000). It now appears that drug toxicity is due, in part, to apoptosis induced by p53 (Komarova and Gudkov,2000).

We can observe several side effects during 5-FU usage, and some side effects are most frequent while others are less common, and it is individual for each person, doses of drugs and way of use. When used as a cream, 5-FU has generally presented very mild side effects.

Commonly, 5-FU may give rise to darkening of skin and nail beds, nausea and vomiting, poor appetite, sores in mouth, lips, or throat, hair loss or thinning, diarrhea, brittle nails, increased sensitivity to sun, dry, flaky, and cracking skin.

5-FU also may temporary increase risk of drop in the number of blood cells (platelet, red and white blood cell count) with bigger risk of infection and tiredness and breathlessness.

Less commonly, it can raise darkening and hardening of veins used for giving the drug, headache, weakness, muscle aches, and rarely can provoke trouble walking, trouble forming words, and poor coordination, irritated eyes, increased tears, watering eyes, blurred vision, heart problems, confusion, tingling, numbness, or swelling in the hands and feet, and severe allergic reaction.

As may occur with an interaction among drugs and supplements, we must be careful when to administrate 5-FU in addition to them.

The mean drugs that present interactions with 5-FU, and increase the risk of side effects are: leucovorin, warfarin, ticlopidine, clopidogrel, vitamin E, and non-steroidal anti-inflammatory drugs (NSAIDs) such as aspirin, ibuprofen, naproxen and many others. So we must remember that many cold, flu, fever, and headache remedies contain aspirin or ibuprofen.

It is also known that drug levels of phenytoin and fosphenytoin may be increased by fluorouracil, and have its actions powered.

Some others conditions must be carefully observed in the case of 5-FU use such as risk of trombosis, once cancer may increase the risk of developing a blood clot, and chemotherapy may increase this risk further, using other medicines must be carefully observed since some medicines, complementary therapies and herbal drugs may be harmful when in addition to 5-FU.

Women may experience amenorrhoea but this may only be temporary. However, male fertility as well as female fertility may be compromised because there is a risk that the child may be affected if pregnancy occurs during chemotherapy or after treatment, so it is important to use effective contraception while taking 5-FU for at least a few months afterwards.

5-FU-related toxicities usually include hematological, digestive and cutaneous features. Additionally, 5-FU has been described as being potentially neurotoxic in patients, but these side effects are quite rare in clinical practice.

Neurotoxicity may include drowsiness, acute confusion plus dysarthria confusion and signs of metabolic encephalopathy (Cordier et al., 2011)

Another important side effect of the chemotherapy, if not the most important, is the cardiotoxicity, and that depends on many different factors related to the drug itself and to the individual patient. Understanding these factors may help to reduce the occurrence or severity of cardiovascular side effects. The dose of the drug administered during each session, cumulative dose, schedule of delivery, route of administration, combination of drugs given, and sequence of administration of these drugs are some important drug-related factors to consider. Patient-related factors include age, previous cardiovascular disease, radiation therapy, metabolic abnormalities, and hypersensitivity to the drugs given. Knowing the risk factors for chemotherapy-induced cardiovascular complication can help to focus preventive efforts to reduce cardiotoxicity (Yeh et al. 2004) Monitoring for other anti-cancer drug–related cardiotoxic effects such as arrhythmias, ischemic cardiac events, and pericardial disease should be planned and specially tailored for each therapeutic protocol according to which anti-cancer agents are prescribed. Cardiac tests such as electrocardiography, rest and stress myocardial perfusion imaging, and troponin levels can be used to monitor ischemic cardiac complications. Twenty-four–hour Holter monitoring can be very helpful in detecting and evaluating suspected arrhythmias. Echocardiography has emerged as the test of choice for the non-invasive evaluation of cardiac disease as related to cancer therapy. This tool is essential in the evaluation of LV systolic and diastolic function, pericardial disease, and detailed evaluation of valvular heart disease. Doppler echocardiography can also be used to assess hemodynamic status, including the presence of pulmonary hypertension (Yeh et al. 2004)

In patients with chemotherapy-induced cardiomyopathy, a decrease in B-type natriuretic peptide (BNP) levels after dobutamine stress echocardiography correlated with the presence of contractile reserve. This finding also correlated with long-term improvement in LV systolic function and New York Heart Association class rating when patients were given β-blockers and angiotensin-converting enzyme (ACE) inhibitors (Tong et al. 2004)

Much cardiac toxicity can be managed best by removing the offending agent. Unfortunately, in the case of newly developed left ventricular (LV) dysfunction, chemotherapy may not be the only explanation for the reduced function, and thus all possible reversible causes should be investigated. In patients with cancer, ischemia is still a reversible cause of LV dysfunction. Cardiac reserve and subsequent improvement after aggressive CHF-based therapy can be predicted by results from dobutamine stress echocardiography (Tong et al., 2004)

More importantly, once therapy is established, it may need to be continued because withdrawal of therapy in some patients has been associated with serious adverse events (Lenihan et al., 2003)

5-fluorouracil (5-FU) has also been responsible for cardiotoxic effects and the most common among them is the ischemic syndrome (Gradishar and Vokes, 1990), which varies clinically from angina pectoris to acute MI. The ischemia is usually reversible on cessation of the 5-FU and implementation of anti-ischemic medical therapy. Ischemia can occur in patients without underlying coronary artery disease (CAD) (incidence, 1.1%), but the incidence is higher in patients with CAD (4.5%) (Labianca et al., 1982).

Important points for observing when 5-FU is used are that side effects may be mild or more severe, and may get better or worse through your course of treatment, or more side effects may develop as the course goes on. These response variations are dependent of how many times the drug was used before, general patient health, amount of drug dose applied and if other drugs are being used in association.

REFERENCES

Albert, J.M,. Buzdar, A.U., Guzman, R., et al. Prospective randomized trial of 5-fluorouracil, doxorubicin, and cyclophosphamide (FAC) versus paclitaxel and FAC (TFAC) in patients with operable breast cancer: impact of taxane chemotherapy on locoregional control. *Breast Cancer Res. Treat.* 2011;128(2):421-7.

Arango, D., Corner, G.A., Wadler, S., et al. c-Myc/p53 interaction determines sensitivity of human colon carcinoma cells to 5-fluorouracil in vitro and in vivo. *Cancer Res.* 2001; 61:4910–5.

Batista, C.S., Atallah, Á.N., Saconato, H., da Silva, E.M.K. 5-FU for genital warts in non-immunocompromised individuals. Cochrane Database of Systematic Reviews 2010, Issue 4. Art. No.: CD006562. DOI: 10.1002 /14651858. CD006562.pub2.

Berlin, J. Second-Line Therapy in Colorectal Cancer. *Oncology.* 2000:14(12Suppl11): 21-6.

Cancer Research UK. http://www.cancerresearchuk.org/

Cordier, P.Y., Nau, A., Ciccolini, J., et al. 5-FU-induced neurotoxicity in cancer patients with profound DPD deficiency syndrome: a report of two cases. *Cancer Chemother. Pharmacol.* 2011;68(3):823-6.

Dyment, P.G. Human Papillomavirus Infection: Reprint from State of the Art Reviews. *Adolescent Medicine*.1996;7.

Gradishar, W.J., Vokes, E.E. 5-Fluorouracil cardiotoxicity: a critical review. *Ann. Oncol.* 1990;1:409–14.

Johnstone, R.W., Ruefli, A.A., Lowe, S.W. Apoptosis: A Link between Cancer Genetics and Chemotherapy. *Cell.* 2002;108(25):153–64.

Komarova, E.A., Gudkov, A.V. Suppression of p53: a new approach to overcome side effects of anti-tumor therapy. *Biochemistry.* 2000; 65:41–8.

Labianca, R., Beretta, G., Clerici, M., et al. Cardiac toxicity of 5-fluorouracil: a study on 1083 patients. *Tumori.* 1982;68:505–10.

Lenihan, D.J., Tong, A.T., Woods, M., et al. Withdrawal of ACE-inhibitors and beta-blockers in chemotherapy induced heart failure leads to severe adverse cardiovascular events. *Circulation.* 2003;108 (suppl IV):665.

Meta-analysis Group in Cancer. Efficacy of intravenous-continuous infusion of fluorouracil compared with bolus administration in advanced colorectal cancer. *J. Clin. Oncol.* 1998;16(1):301-8.

Milano, G, Chamorey, A.L. Clinical pharmacokinetics of 5-fluorouracil with consideration of chronopharmacokinetics. *Chronobiol. Int.* 2002;19(1):177-89.

Moertel, C.G. Chemotherapy for colorectal cancer. *N. Engl. J. Med.* 1994;330: 1136-42.

Nair, K.L, Jagadeeshan, S, Nair, S.A. et al. Biological evaluation of 5-fluorouracil nanoparticles for cancer chemotherapy and its dependence on the carrier, PLGA. *Int. J. Nanomedicine.* 2011;6:1685-97.

National Cancer Institute (NCI). http://www.cancer.gov/

O'Connell, M.J., Mailliard, J.A., Kahn, M.J., et al. Controlled trial of fluorouracil and low-dose leucovorin given for 6 months as postoperative adjuvant therapy for colon cancer. *J. Clin. Oncol.* 1997;15:246-50.

Shiratori, Claudia; Akemi, Hoyama, Érika; Schellini, lvana Artioli; Padovani, Carlos Roberto. Infiltração de 5-fluorouracil no pré-operatório do pterígio. *Arq. Bras. Oftalmol.* [serial on the Internet]. 2003 Aug [cited 2012 Feb 27] ; 66(4): 499-503. Available from: http://www.scielo.br/scielo.php?script =sci_arttextandpid=S0004-27492003000400020andlng=en. http://dx.doi.org/10.1590/S0004-27492003000400020.

Silvana, A., et al. Uso do 5-fluorouracil no intra-operatório da cirurgia do pterígio. *Arq. Bras. Oftalmol.* [online]. 2000, vol.63, n.2 [cited 2012-02-27], pp. 111-114. Available from: <http://www.scielo.br/scielo.php?scrip =sci _arttextandpid=S0004-27492000000200003andlng=enandnrm=iso>. ISSN 0004-2749. http://dx.doi.org/10.1590/S0004-27492000000200003.

Tong, A.T., Lenihan, D., Divakaran, V., et al. B-type natriuretic peptide is a biochemical predictor of myocardial contractile reserve during dobutamine stress echocardiogram. *J. Am. Coll. Cardiol.* 2004;43:173(A).

Tonon, L.M., Silvia Secoli, S.R., Caponero, R. Câncer colorretal: uma revisão da abordagem terapêutica com bevacizumabe [A review of bevacizumab and its use in colorectal cancer]. *Rev. bras. cancerol.* 2007;53(2): 173-82.

Wilkes, G.M. Therapeutic options in the managment of colon cancer. *Clin. J. Onco. Nurs.* 2005;9(1):31-44.

Wolmark, N., Rockette, H., Mamounas, E., et al. Clinical trial to assess the relative efficacy of fluorouracil and leucovorin, fluorouracil and levamisole, and fluorouracil, leucovorin, and levamisole in patients with Dukes' and carcinoma of the colon: results from National Surgical Adjuvant Breast and Bowel Project C-04. *J. Clin. Oncol.* 1999; 17 (11):

Valezi, Vanessa Grandi; Schellini Silvana, Artioli; Viveiros Magda Massae Hata; Padovani, Carlos Roberto. Segurança e efetividade no tratamento do pterígio usando infiltração de 5-fluoruracila no intraoperatório. *Arq. Bras. Oftalmol.* [serial on the Internet]. 2009 Apr [cited 2012 Feb 27] ; 72(2): 169-173. Available from: http://www.scielo.br/scielo.php?script =sci_arttextandpid =S0004-27492009000200007andlng=en.   http://dx.doi.org/10.1590/S0004-27492009000200007.

Yeh, E.T., Tong, A.T., Lenihan, D.J., et al. Cardiovascular complications of cancer therapy: diagnosis, pathogenesis, and management. *Circulation.* 2004;109:3122-31. DOI 10.1161/01.CIR.0000133187.74800.B9

In: Fluorouracil
Editors: A. Longinho and S. Dobreiro

ISBN: 978-1-62081-970-8
© 2012 Nova Science Publishers, Inc.

Chapter V

LONG-TERM RESULTS OF NEEDLE REVISION AND 'OVER THE FLAP 5-FLUOROURACIL APPLICATION' IN THE MANAGEMENT OF BLEB FAILURE

Ismet Durak, Zeynep Ozbek, Aylin Yaman, Meltem Soylev and Güray Çingil*
Dokuz Eylül University School of Medicine,
Department of Ophthalmology, Izmir, Turkey

ABSTRACT

Sixty-five eyes of 61 consecutive patients with an intraocular pressure (IOP) over 21 mmHg; without bleb or with a thick, flat bleb after the second postoperative week following trabeculectomy were enrolled in the study. Needle revision was performed initially using a 26-gauge tuberculin syringe containing 5 mg (0.2ml) 5-Fluorouracil (5-FU) within a period of two weeks to 6 months postoperatively after unsuccessful digital massage and/or laser suture-lysis. 5-FU injection was not performed when bleb formation was observed during needling. In case of no bleb formation, 5-FU was injected subconjunctivally over the scleral flap area and repeated weekly for a

---

* Address of corresponding author: Dr. Ismet Durak, Mithatpasa cad. 259/8, 35340 Balcova Izmir, Turkey, Phone: 90 232 2597256, Facsimile: 90 232 277 43 98, E-mail: hdurak@kordon.deu.edu.tr.

maximum of six times until a functioning bleb was maintained. Needle revision was successful in 18 of 65 eyes (27.7%) as an initial procedure and 12 eyes (18.5%) maintained success. Fifty-three eyes (81.5%) had 5-FU injection since needle revision did not provide bleb formation (47 eyes) or did not maintain initial success (6 eyes). Mean intraocular pressure was 28.2+4.9 mmHg (range: 22-41) before any intervention and decreased to 20.4+4.8 mmHg (range: 10-35) after a mean follow-up of 32.2 months and the difference was statistically significant (p<0.001). Mean IOP after needle revision in 18 eyes was 18.8+4.9 (range: 8-29) and 16.2+3.8 mmHg in twelve out of 18 patients that maintained success. Mean IOP after the last 5-FU injection was 21.2+4.6 mmHg (range: 12-35). The mean number of 5-FU injections was 2.4 (range:1-6). During a mean follow-up of 32.2 months (range: 1-56 months) three eyes (4.6%) had diffuse corneal punctate epitheliopathy lasting for 2-3 weeks and subconjuctival hemorrhage was seen in 10 eyes (15.4%). The drug leaked into the anterior chamber causing no complications in one eye and immediate superior limbal vascularization of the cornea was observed in one eye. Needle revision and/or subconjuctival 5-FU injection over the flap area is a safe and relatively efficient approach with low rate of minor complications in the management of bleb failure in long term as well as in the early postoperative period.

Keywords: Bleb dysfunction, bleb failure, fluorouracil, glaucoma, glaucoma surgery, needle-revision

INTRODUCTION

Since filtering cicatrix was first described as a surgical treatment for glaucoma, many different filtering procedures have been performed to establish a fistula between the anterior chamber and the subconjunctival space [1]. Trabeculectomy originally described by Cairns in 1968 has been the prototype glaucoma filtering procedure ever since [2]. Despite modifications of the technique and evolution of some new trends in glaucoma surgery lately, trabeculectomy is the golden standard according to many surgeons. Unlike many types of surgery in which complete healing of tissue with restoration of normal architecture would be a desirable outcome, glaucoma surgery aims at incomplete healing to allow aqueous humor to drain in an alternative way. Since completely healed trabeculectomy means a failed trabeculectomy, the goal is to maintain long-term filtration [2].

Success rates after filtration surgery are reported between 67% and 94% in the literature however the longer the follow-up, the lower success values are. First reports of trabeculectomy give higher success ratios such as in Ferguson and Macdonald' s study [3] which reported 87% success in a series of 31 eyes of 25 patients while Schwartz et al had 92% success on 33 eyes during one-year follow-up [4]. D' Ermo et al stated that complete success was achieved in 71% of their cases during a follow-up of 5 years [5]. Another study by Inaba [6] was comprised of 427 Japanese patients and had an overall success rate of 75% in controlling the intraocular pressure (IOP) below 21 mmHg. In 344 eyes followed more than 1 year, the IOP distribution showed that the IOP was between 14 and 19 mmHg in 47% of the eyes, and in only 2.3% was the IOP lower than 10 mmHg.

Another point to consider about the results of glaucoma surgery is that success is higher in primary open angle glaucoma than narrow angle, pseudoexfoliative or secondary glaucomas. Gressel and friends [7] showed that success rate in primary glaucomas (29/39, 74%) was considerably higher than in secondary glaucomas (24/50, 48%) or in developmental glaucomas (6/17, 35%). Only one (9%) of 11 trabeculectomies performed for neovascular glaucoma was successful.

Also it has been shown that chronic use of topical antiglaucoma agents has a deterious effect on the success of filtration surgery. Especially long-term treatment with adrenergic agonists results in morphologic changes on the conjunctiva and Tenon's capsule like subclinical inflammation associated with an increased number of fibroblasts [8,9]. The greatest adverse effect was reportedly induced by triple topical therapy consisting of a beta-blocker, a miotic and an adrenergic agonist [10]. This knowledge led some surgeons to suggest that glaucoma surgery should be as initial therapy [2].

The success of glaucoma surgery unfortunately has been limited by postoperative scarring. Scarring most commonly occurs at the level of the episclera leading to flap fibrosis and eventual bleb failure. Whereas intraoperative precautions like control of bleeding and postoperative management such as anti-inflammatory agents target at reducing fibroblastic activity, they are eventually insufficient to prevent scarring for the long-term [2]. Many attempts have been made to modulate wound healing and bleb function after filtration surgery. Topical and systemic corticosteroids, digital ocular compression and focal compression, laser suture-lysis, releasable sutures, tissue plasminogen activator, laser internal revision, transconjunctival needle revision, beta-irradiation and use of antimetabolites are different modalities advocated to restore bleb function [11]. The two most commonly used antimetabolites in glaucoma surgery are 5-Fluorouracil and Mitomycin C.

Five-fluorouracil (5-FU) is a chemotherapeutic agent that specifically mediates its antiproliferative effect by antagonizing pyrimidine metabolism. It effectively inhibits fibroblast growth and function. It is particularly useful as an adjunct to inhibit wound healing during and after glaucoma filtration surgery by improving long-term bleb function [2,13]. Traditionally, 5-FU applications are performed in the early postoperative period, most often starting on the second or third postoperative day in a quadrant 90 or 180 degrees away from the filtration site in order to avoid any undesired complication like drug penetration to the anterior chamber, bleb necrosis or infection [2, 13, 14]. Needle revision and 5-FU injections are generally performed as separate procedures. In this study, we performed needle revision alone and together with "modified" subconjunctival 5-FU injections directly over the filtration site, starting after the second postoperative week. The purpose of the study was to overcome early and mid-term bleb failure and to evaluate the results.

MATERIALS AND METHODS

Sixty-five eyes of 61 consecutive patients who underwent trabeculectomy between February 1993 and December 2002 in the Department of Ophthalmology Dokuz Eylul University School of Medicine, Izmir, Turkey were included in the study. Inclusion criteria were no bleb or a thick, flat bleb together with an IOP over 21 mm Hg after second postoperative week. The group consisted of 39 male and 22 female patients.

Each patient underwent a thorough ophthalmological examination before deciding surgery and gave informed consent. Preoperative evaluation included determination of the best corrected visual acuity by using Snellen chart, slit-lamp biomicroscopy of the anterior segment, determination of the intraocular pressure by Goldmann applanation tonometry, examination of the anterior chamber angle by gonioscopy, assessment of the optic nerve cupping using Goldmann three-mirror lens or 78 D lens and testing of visual fields by standard white-white Humphrey automated perimetry.

The decision criteria for trabeculectomy were progression in optic disc cupping or visual field deterioration confirmed by two different observers and intraocular pressure levels over 21 mm Hg despite maximal antiglaucoma therapy during at least two consecutive control visits. Surgery was performed by 4 different surgeons using a standardized technique: A fornix-based conjunctival dissection, slight cauterization of the surgical field, preparation of a triangular or rectangular scleral flap, excision of 1 x 3 mm trabecular tissue and peripheral iridectomy. The scleral flap was closed using one or two 10/0 nylon sutures ant the conjunctiva was apposed using separate 8/0 polyglactin sutures. Tenon excision was performed when needed. No antimetabolites were used during surgery. Patients who had undergone trabeculectomy combined with cataract extraction or any other concurrent or previous intraocular surgery were not included in the study. All patients were treated postoperatively with topical steroids and antibiotics six times a day and cycloplegics three times a day for one week. Cycloplegics were stopped and the steroids were gradually tapered in the following weeks. Patients were evaluated by weekly follow-up visits. Visual acuity, biomicroscopic evaluation of the anterior segment and the flap area, intraocular pressure levels, examination of the fundus were performed in each visit. In case of an intraocular pressure below 10mmHg, B-mode orbital ultrasound examination was done in order to rule out choroidal or retinal detachment.

If no bleb was observed and the intraocular pressure was over 20 mmHg at the first two postoperative visits, Argon laser suture-lysis (Zeiss, spot size: 50 microns/ power: 400-800 mw/ duration: 0.2 sec) using a Hoskin's lens was performed in the second postoperative week and then digital massage was applied in order to provide filtering. In case of persisting high IOP and no filtering bleb after two weeks despite digital massage and suture-lysis, needling was done with a tuberculin syringe containing 5-FU *(250mg/ml, Biosyn, Biosynarzneimittel GmbH Hellbach, Germany)* under topical anesthesia in outpatient basis, The technique was as follows: A 26-gauge needle was introduced subconjunctivally from the temporal quadrant and moved to the bleb site, while elevating the scleral flap slightly. Fluorouracil injection was not performed if bleb formation took place during needle revision. In eyes that bleb formation was not observed after needling, 5 mg (0.2 ml) 5-FU was injected subconjunctivally over the scleral flap just after needling. Then the cornea was irrigated copiously with at least 50 ml sterile saline solution. The eye was patched for 24 hours and prophylactic topical antibiotic treatment was given if the patient was not already on standard postoperative treatment regimen. Repeated weekly doses of 5-FU were given according to the IOP value and the biomicroscopic appearance of the bleb site on the 3-5th day of application until a filtering bleb was maintained. The total dose used varied from patient to patient with a maximum of six applications.

Complete success was defined as an IOP of 21 mmHg or less without any medication and relative success was defined as an IOP of 21 mmHg or less with one anti-glaucoma medication. Intraocular pressure values before and after needle revision and 5-FU application were compared using Student's t- test for paired samples. $p < 0.05$ was accepted as significant.

RESULTS

A total of 65 eyes of 61 patients (39 males and 22 females) were included in the study. Mean age of the patients was 66.5 years at the time of surgery (range: 48-82 years). Eleven eyes had (16.9%) pseudoexfoliative glaucoma, 4 eyes (6.1%) had narrow angle glaucoma, while 50 eyes (76.9%) had uncontrolled primary open angle glaucoma (POAG) despite maximum antiglaucoma medication.

Eighteen out of 65 eyes (27.7%) underwent needle revision only as an initial procedure since bleb formation was observed during needling and success was maintained in 12 eyes with needle revision (18.5%). After needle-revision, 6 eyes remained under 21 mmHg without any glaucoma medication; 6 eyes were controlled with one glaucoma medication. 5-FU was applied later to the remaining 6 eyes besides the 47 eyes (total 53 eyes) that no bleb formation occurred after needle revision. The methodology of the study procedure is summarized as a flow chart in Figure-1. Table-1 shows the mean intraocular pressure values of all groups before and after all interventions and Table-2 gives the complete, relative and total success ratios after needle revision and 5-FU injections. There was a statistically significant difference between baseline and final IOP for all eyes.

Thirteen eyes (20%) restored bleb function after only one injection of subconjunctival 5-FU; nine eyes (13.8%) needed 2 injections, six eyes (9.2%) needed three injections and the remaining 25 eyes (38.5%) required more than three injections to maintain bleb function. Mean intraocular pressure was 28.2+4.9 mmHg (range: 22-41) before any intervention and decreased to 20.4+4.8 mmHg (range: 10-35) after a mean follow-up of 32.2 months and the difference was statistically significant (p<0.001). Mean intraocular pressure after needle revision in 18 eyes was 18.8+4.9 (range: 8-29) and 16.2+3.8 mmHg in twelve out of 18 patients that maintained success. Mean IOP after the last 5-FU injection was 21.2+4.6 mmHg (range: 12-35). Mean number of 5-FU applications was 2.4 (range 1 to 6). The earliest application was at the second postoperative week while the latest was at 6 months after the surgery (mean: 2.1 months). During a mean follow-up of 32.2 months (range 1 to 56 months), 3 eyes (4.6%) had diffuse corneal punctate epitheliopathy after 5-FU application lasting for 2-3 weeks and subconjunctival hemorrhage took place in 10 eyes (15.4%). Corneal punctate staining subsided completely with topical lubricant therapy and subconjunctival hemorrhage resolved spontaneously without any additional intervention. 5-FU leaked into the anterior chamber in one case. The drug was observed to stream down slowly in an oily fashion on biomicroscopy after the injection but this did not cause any complication or anterior segment reaction. Interestingly, corneal vascularization at the superotemporal limbus was observed in one eye two weeks after 5-FU application but no anterior chamber reaction was noted. (This patient was not the same with whom the drug penetrated the anterior chamber) No other complications such as choroidal detachment, hypotony maculopathy, bleb necrosis or late endophthalmitis were observed related to the needle revision or 5-FU injection.

Table 1. The mean IOP of all groups before and after interventions

	Initial IOP	**Final IOP**
Total	28.2±4.7 (22-41)	18.8±4.9
NR success (12)	26.6±3.5 (23-35)	16.2±3.8
5-FU (53)	28.0±4.9 (22-41)	21.2±4.6

NR: Needle revision.
5-FU: 5-Fluorouracil.

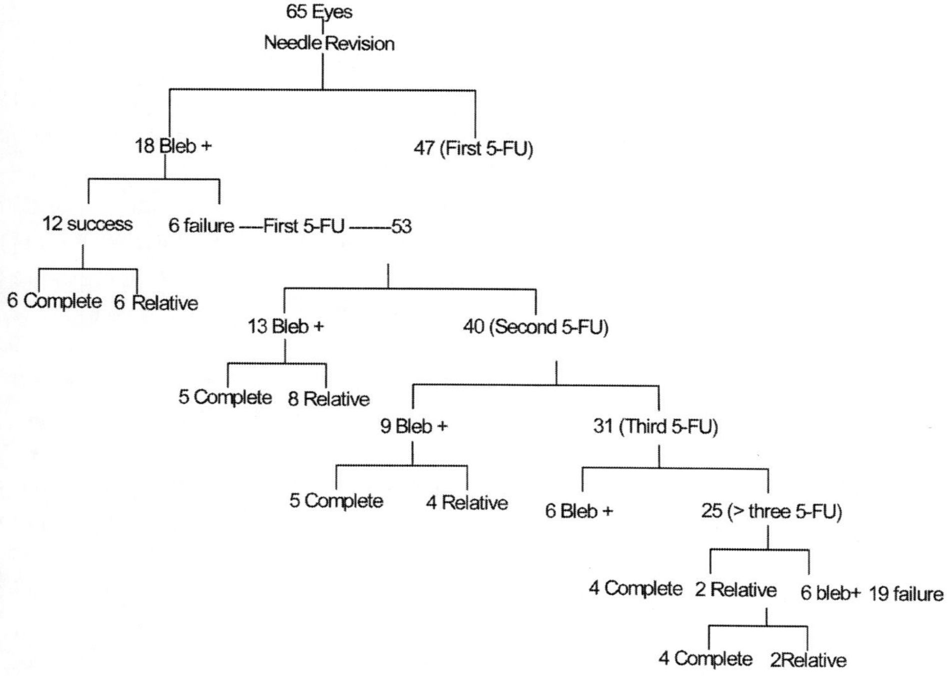

Figure 1. Flow Chart summarizing the technique.

**Table-2. The complete, relative and total success after
needle revision and 5-FU injection**

	Complete success	Relative success	Total success	Cumulative
	n (%)	n (%)	n (%)	n (%)
NR (65)	6 (9.2%)	6 (9.2%)	12(18.4%)	12 (18.4%)
First 5-FU (53)	5(9.4%)	8 (15.09%)	13 (24.5%)	25 (38.5%)
Second 5-FU (40)	5(12.5%)	4 (10%)	9(22.5%)	34 (52.3%)
Third 5-FU (31)	4 (12.9%)	2 (6.5%)	6(19.4%)	40 (61.5%)
>3 times 5-FU (25)	4 (16%)	2 (8%)	6 (24%)	46 (70.7%)
Failure			19 (29.2%)	19 (29.2%)
Final success	24 (36.9%)	16 (33.8%)	46 (70.7%)	

DISCUSSION

Successful glaucoma filtering surgery is characterized by the passage of aqueous humor from the anterior chamber to the subconjunctival space, which results in the formation of a filtering functional bleb; an alternative way for the aqeous to leave the eye [13,14]. Success rates after filtration surgery are reported as between 67% and 94% during five years' follow-up in different reports. [1] However, the success of glaucoma surgery is limited by postoperative scarring leading to flap fibrosis and eventual bleb failure which still remains to be a common concern.

The initial process in the natural wound healing response is inflammation and coagulation, leading to a cascade of biological events including cellular, hormonal and growth factor related reactions [2]. Type and duration of glaucoma, chronic use of multiple topical antiglaucomatous medications, previous surgery, ocular inflammatory diseases, age and race are among the pre-existing factors affecting this response.

Intraoperative manipulations like control of bleeding, gentle handling and careful dissection, excision of Tenon also play a role on the surgical outcome [2]. As for the postoperative modulation of healing, topical corticosteroids are the mainstay of postoperative treatment regimen following ocular surgery whereas systemic steroids which did not provide any additional benefit for glaucoma surgery [15] are seldom used. Inhibition of inflammation and wound healing by corticosteroids is mediated via suppression of leukocyte concentration, distribution and function as well as their effects on vascular permeability. This leads to less leakage of serum and clotting factors and hence formation of clot and fibrin [2].

Intraoperative application of antifibrotics is a commonly preferred option to help diminish postoperative fibrosis. Digital ocular compression and focal compression, laser suture-lysis, releasable sutures, laser internal revision, transconjunctival needle revision, beta-irradiation are postoperative manipulations which may be performed in an attempt to restore bleb function [11].

Most commonly preferred techniques are intraoperative and postoperative application of antifibrotic agents with or without other postoperative manipulations like needle revision. Mitomycin C and 5-Fluorouracil are used as an adjunct to glaucoma surgery since 1980s.

Mitomycin C is an antibiotic drug which undergoes metabolic activation via reduction into an alkylating agent that cross-links DNA. It is a non cell-cycle specific drug that not only inhibits DNA replication but also mitosis and protein synthesis in fibroblasts and endothelial cells [2].

Five-fluorouracil (5-FU) is a chemotherapeutic agent that specifically mediates its antiproliferative effect by antagonizing pyrimidine metabolism, inhibition of DNA synthesis and ultimately cell death. It has been demonstrated to be a very effective inhibitor of fibroblast growth and function. It is a cell-cycle specific drug and selectivelly affects actively replicating cells [16].

Khaw et al compared the effects on fibroblast outgrowth following 5-minute applications of 5-FU (50 mg/ml), Mitomycin C (0.4 mg/ml) or distilled water in rabbits undergoing full-thickness glaucoma-filtering surgery. They found that fibroblasts cultured from tissue samples obtained from rabbits treated with Mitomycin C still evidenced growth inhibition at 1 month while fibroblasts from 5-FU-treated rabbits demonstrated full recovery of growth arrest after 7 days [17].

Smith et al performed cell culture experiments using Mouse 3t3 fibroblasts and capillary endothelial cells exposed to varying concentrations of 5-FU and Mitomycin C. They found that both cell types were susceptible to Mitomycin C, fibroblasts were far more sensitive to 5-FU than endothelial cells and concluded that 5-FU is toxic to fibroblasts but spares endothelial cells whereas Mitomycin C is cytotoxic to both types [18]. Intraoperative application of Mitomycin C renders high success ratios however is also associated with development of potentially serious side effects like thin-walled avascular blebs and related late onset bleb leaks and endophthalmitis besides severe hypotony causing choroidal detachment and maculopathy [19]. Therefore Mitomycin C is preserved for high risk patients like those with uveitis or neovascular glaucoma. Intraoperative 5-FU yields similiar or slightly lower success ratios when compared to Mitomycin C in low risk patients with relatively low rate of complications. However, success ratios appear to diminish with longer follow-up since fibrosis continues to occur even in eyes with established successful early filtration [20].

At that point, postoperative subconjunctival injections of 5-FU have been reported to increase the success of trabeculectomy, to decrease the IOP and the postoperative glaucoma medication. According to the Fluorouracil Filtering Surgery Group's one year follow-up results, 5-FU injections in the first two postoperative weeks, results in a statistically significant IOP fall especially in the second and fourth postoperative weeks [13]. After one-year follow-up, failure rates were 27% in the 5-FU group versus 50% in the standard treatment group. Therefore, the Fluorouracil Filtering Surgery Group recommends the use of subconjunctival 5-FU injection after trabeculectomy in eyes with uncontrolled glaucoma and poor prognoses, specifically for pseudophakic or aphakic glaucoma and unsuccessful filtering surgery. Most of the bleb failures are at the episcleral level due to fibrovascular regeneration. Needling and 5-FU injection may alter fibrovascular regeneration and aqueous humour outflow.

The effectiveness of trabeculectomy with adjunctive low dose 5-fluorouracil (5-FU) as the initial surgical procedure in uncomplicated glaucoma was evaluated retrospectively in a consecutive series of 52 patients (mean follow-up, 18.6 +/- 11.7 months) and 74 control subjects. The cumulative 2-year success (intraocular pressure [IOP] less than 21 mmHg) was 100% in the 5-FU group and 78.9% in the control group The 5-FU group had a mean postoperative IOP of 12.5 +/- 4.6 mmHg versus 17.4 +/- 5.7 mmHg in the control group at 2-year follow-up. Antiglaucoma medications were required in 5.8% of patients in the 5-FU group and in 41.9% of controls within 2 years [21].

In a study by Watanabe et al, the records of 205 eyes of 168 patients were retrospectively reviewed. A life table analysis and a comparison was made between patients who had trabeculectomy with and without subconjunctival 5-FU. The success rate at 30 months after trabeculectomy with 5-FU therapy was considerably higher in primary open-angle glaucoma at 93.6% (72.7%), secondary glaucoma at 88.9% (72.4%), and refractory glaucoma at 72.2% (32.5%) with (or without) the use of ocular hypotensive drops when compared with historical control groups treated without 5-FU (60.0% (41.7%), 35.5% (24.0%), and 18.0% (8.0%), respectively) [22].

Another Japanese study reported long-term results in a total of 362 eyes of 263 glaucoma patients with the postoperative follow-up of 1-9 years. The probability of successful intraocular pressure (IOP) control at the 5-year point of the continuing follow-up was calculated by the life-table method of Kaplan-Meier. The eyes that had undergone trabeculectomy with postoperative injections of 5-FU (5-FU group) included 165 eyes with primary open-angle glaucoma

(POAG), 38 eyes with secondary glaucoma (SG) and 60 eyes with refractory glaucoma. The eyes that had undergone trabeculectomy without postoperative 5-FU (control group) included 46 eyes with POAG, 31 eyes with SG and 22 eyes with refractory glaucoma. The surgical techniques and postoperative care were virtually identical between the two groups, except that the control group did not receive the postoperative 5-FU. The total amount of 5-FU given to each case averaged 36.5, 36.0 and 49.5 mg for POAG, SG and refractory glaucoma, respectively. At the 5-year follow-up point, the probability of maintaining IOP control below 21 mmHg with or without medication in the 5-FU group was 92.5% for POAG, 87.4% for SG and 57.5% for refractory glaucoma; while without medication the probability was 58.2, 54.8 and 27.8%, respectively. The probability of IOP control below 16 mmHg with or without medication in the 5-FU group was 77.9% for POAG, 66.8% for SG and 26.9% for refractory glaucoma; without medication the probability was 55.2, 49.8 and 24.5%, respectively. In the control group, the corresponding probability for each type of glaucoma was much lower than that in the 5-FU group, and the probability for IOP control below 16 mm Hg was 0.12% at the 5-year follow-up point. In the 5-FU group, the mean postoperative IOP in successfully treated eyes remained at about 12 mmHg throughout the first 5 years of the follow-up period. There was no significant difference in incidence of postoperative complications between the 5-FU and control groups, except that corneal epithelial defect was noted in 38.8% of the eyes in the 5-FU group. No late complications related to the use of postoperative 5-FU were observed [23].

Greenfield and co-authors used needling and 5-FU injection in the inferior fornix (when necessary) for failed bleb after trabeculectomy with Mitomycin-C and found a success rate of 73% in 63 eyes [24]. They found that adjunctive use of 5-FU at the time of needling increases the success rate. Pederson and Smith performed needling in 13 cases and reported successful results in 9 cases (69%) [25]. But 6 of 9 patients required anti-glaucoma medications for success. Ewing and Stamper used 5-FU with needle revision in 12 patients with failed blebs [26]. Seven patients received 5-FU injections up to 11 times. Total and complete success rates were 91.6% and 63.6% respectively. Although they did not find a statistically significant difference for 5-FU injection, their clinical impression suggested a favourable effect. Shin et al reported 80% success rate after needle revision and 5-FU injection in 30 cases [27]. But complete success rate was only 16.7% in their study. Mardelli et al applied Mitomycin-C and needling after a mean of 4.1 years for failed filtration surgery [28]. They reported that Mitomycin needle revision is an extremely effective way to revive failed filtration surgery. Goldenfeld et al applied subconjunctival 5mg 5-FU to the 32 patients with uncontrolled phakic glaucoma in the first two weeks after trabeculectomy and compared their results with a control group of 30 patients [29]. After a minimum follow-up of one year, IOP and the number of glaucoma medications were significantly lower in the 5-FU group. IOP was 20mmHg or lower in 94% of the 5-FU group it was 73% in the control group.

But in a prospective randomized study of 25 eyes, Costa et al reported 90% success with medical treatment alone versus 7.1% success with needle revision in cases with bleb encapsulation [30]. They observed that the typical response of a patient undergoing needling was an important IOP reduction during the first week, followed by an abrupt increase in IOP with recurrence of encapsulated bleb. The success rate of needling in our series was 27.7% (18 eyes out of 65) with a mean follow-up of 32.2 months. It is not possible to make an exact comparison of the studies since the patient population, inclusion criteria, drug doses, techniques and success criteria are not the same. Success of needling in some cases lies in mechanical removal of the fibrin plug and/or tearing of tenon encapsulation and maintenance of a patent filtration site by continuous flow of aqueous with its inhibitory effects.

Traditionally, 5-FU application is started in the immediate postoperative period and it is completed by the end of the second postoperative week. Also subconjunctival injections of 5-FU are commonly performed 90 to 180 degrees away from the bleb site. We preferred to inject over the bleb area since injection of 5-FU on the bleb site probably provides higher concentration of the drug, which in turn provides more anti-fibroblastic effect. Primary concern in injecting the antimetabolite 180° away from the bleb site is to avoid drug entrance to the anterior chamber. In our series, 5-FU was injected to eyes without bleb formation during needle revision, so the risk of direct communication of the drug with anterior chamber was supposed to be absent or very low. Although 5-FU oozed accidentally into the anterior chamber in one eye; no anterior segment reaction or corneal endothelial dysfunction was observed probably because the drug' s effect is limited on actively proliferating cells [31,32]. Mazey et al reported significant but reversible corneal edema after 5-FU injection for failed trabeculectomy and speculated that the effect of intraocular fluorouracil may be related to alkaline properties of the solution, to its antimetabolite effect or combination of both or to other unidentified mechanism [33].

Several complications known to be associated with needle revision and 5-FU injection are wound leak, choroidal effusion, shallow anterior chamber, bleb related endophthalmitis and hypotony maculopathy and suprachoroidal hemorrhage [34,35]. Only complications in our series were diffuse corneal punctate epitheliopathy lasting for 2-3 weeks in 3 eyes (probably due to leaking of

5-FU from the subconjunctival space and inadequate irrigation after injection) and subconjunctival hemorrhage in 10 eyes that multiple 5-FU injections were applied. Ewing and Stamper reported the large epithelial defect in 5 (71.4%) of seven eyes [26]. Goldenfeld et al reported superficial punctate keratopathy in 44% of cases after 5-FU injection [29]. The Fluorouracil filtering study group reported punctate corneal epitheliopathy and corneal epithelial defects in 98% and 64% of cases during the postoperative first two weeks. High rate of punctate keratopathy may be due to inadequate irrigation, diagnostic criteria for punctate keratopathy and number of injections in these studies. Copious irrigation of the eyes after 5-FU injection may prevent corneal complications. Interestingly, immediate superior limbal vascularization of the cornea one week after 5-FU application was observed in one eye but no anterior chamber reaction was noted.A missed small limbal ulser result in such a corneal vascularization at the limbus.

In our series, the goal of IOP of 21 mmHg or less without or with one anti-glaucoma medication was achieved in 70.7% of the 65 eyes. In conclusion, combined needle revision and/or subconjunctival 5-FU applications at the bleb site is a safe and relatively efficient approach to increase the success with low rate of complications in the mid term bleb failure after trabeculectomy.

REFERENCES

[1]   Skuta GL, Parrish II RK. Wound healing in glaucoma filtering surgery. Major Review. *Survey of Ophthalmology* 1987; 32(3): 149-170.

[2]   Lama PJ, Fechtner RD. Antifibrotics and wound healing in glaucoma surgery. *Survey of Ophthalmology* 2003; 48: 314-346.

[3]   Ferguson JG Jr, Macdonald R. Trabeculectomy. *South Med J.* 1977; 70(1): 73-4.

[4]   Schwartz PL, Ackerman J, Beards J, Wesseley Z, Goodstein S, Ballen PH.Further experience with trabeculectomy. *Ann Ophthalmol.* 1976 Feb; 8(2): 207-17.

[5]   D'Ermo F, Bonomi L, Doro D. A critical analysis of the long-term results of trabeculectomy. *Am J Ophthalmol.* 1979 Nov; 88(5): 829-35.

[6]   Inaba Z. Long-term results of trabeculectomy in the Japanese: an analysis by life-table method. *Jpn J Ophthalmol.* 1982; 26(4): 361-73.

[7]   Gressel MG, Heuer DK, Parrish RK 2nd. Trabeculectomy in young patients. *Ophthalmology.* 1984 Oct; 91(10): 1242-6.

[8]   Broadway D, Grierson I, Hitchings R. Adverse effects of topical antiglaucoma medications on the conjunctiva. *Br J Ophthalmol.* 1993; 77: 790-6.

[9]   Sherwood MB, Grierson I, Millar L, Hitchings RA. Long-term morphologic effects of antiglaucoma drugs on the conjunctiva and Tenons capsule in glaucomatous patients. *Ophthalmology* 1989; 96: 327-335.

[10] Broadway DC, Grierson I, O'Brien C, Hitchings RA. Adverse effects of topical antiglaucoma medication II. The outcome of filtration surgery. *Arch Ophthalmol* 1994; 112:1446-1154.

[11] Azuara-Blanco A, Katz LJ. Dysfunctional filtering blebs. Major Review. *Survey of Ophthalmol* 1998; 43(2): 93-126.

[12] Falck FY,Skuta GL, Klein TB. Mitomycin C versus 5-Fluorouracil antimetabolite therapy for glaucoma filtration surgery. *Semin Ophthalmol* 1992; 7: 97.

[13] The Fluorouracil Filtering Study Group. Fluorouracil Filtering Study one-year follow-up. *Am J Ophthalmol* 1989: 108; 625-635.

[14] Michel JW, Liebmann JM, Ritch R. Initial 5-Fluorouracil trabeculectomy in young patients *Ophthalmology* 1992; 99: 7-13.

[15] Sarita RJ, Fellman RL, Spaeth GL et al. Short and long-term effects of postoperative corticosteroids on trabeculectomy. *Ophthalmology* 1985; 92: 938-946.

[16] Jampel HD, Jabs DA, Quigley HA. Trabeculectomy with 5-fluorouracil for adult inflammatory glaucoma. *Am J Ophthalmol* 1990: 109; 168-173.

[17] Khaw PT, Doyle WJ, Sherwood MB et al. Prolonged localized tissue effects from 5-minute exposures to fluorouracil and mitomycin. *Arch Ophthalmol* 1993; 111: 263-267.

[18] Smith S, DAmore PA, Dreyer EB. Comparative toxicity of Mitomycin C and 5-Fluorouracil in vitro. *Am J Ophthalmol* 1994: 118; 332-337.

[19] Greenfield DS, Liebmann JM, Jee J, Ritch R. Late-onset bleb leaks after glaucoma filtering surgery. *Arch Ophthalmol* 1998; 116: 443-7.

[20] Bell RW, Habib NE, O'Brien C. Long-term results and complications after trabeculectomy with a single per-operative application of 5-fluorouracil. *Eye* 1997; 11: 663-71.

[21] Liebmann JM, Ritch R, Marmor M, Nunez J, Wolner B. Initial 5-fluorouracil trabeculectomy in uncomplicated glaucoma. *Ophthalmology.* 1991 Jul;98(7):1036-41.

[22] Watanabe J, Iwata K, Sawaguchi S, Nanba K. Trabeculectomy with 5-fluorouracil. *Acta Ophthalmol* (Copenh). 1991 Aug; 69(4): 455-61.

[23] Araie M, Shoji N, Shirato S, Nakano Y. Postoperative subconjunctival 5-fluorouracil injections and success probability of trabeculectomy in Japanese: results of 5-year follow-up. *Jpn J Ophthalmol.* 1992;36(2):158-68.

[24] Greenfield DS, Miller MP, Suner IJ, Palmberg PF. Needle elevation of the scleral flap for failing filtration blebs after trabeculectomy with Mitomycin C. *Am J Ophthalmol* 1996: 122; 195-200.

[25] Pederson JE, Smith SG. Surgical management of encapsulated filtering blebs. *Ophthalmology* 1985; 92: 955-958.

[26] Ewing RH, Stamper RL. Needle revision with and without 5-Fluorouracil for the treatment of failed filtering blebs. *Am J Ophthalmol* 1990: 110; 254-259.

[27] Shin DH, Juzych MS, Khatana AK et al. Needling revision of failed filtering blebs with adjunctive 5-Fluorouracil. *Ophthalmic Surg* 1993; 24: 242-248.

[28] Mardelli PG, Lederer CM, Murray PL, Pastor SA, Hassanein KM. Slit-lamp needle revision of failed filtering blebs using Mitomycin C. *Ophthalmology* 1996; 103: 1946-1955.

[29] Goldenfeld M, Krupin T, Ruderman JM et al. 5-Fluorouracil in initial trabeculectomy. *Ophthalmology* 1994; 101(6):1024-1029

[30] Costa VP, Correa MM, Kara-Jose N. Needling versus medical treatment in encapsulated blebs. *Ophthalmology* 1997; 104(8):1215-1220.

[31] Khaw PT, Sherwood MB, Mac Kay LD et al. Five minute treatments with Fluorouracil, floxuridine and mitomycin have long-term effects oh human Tenon's capsule fibroblasts. *Arch Ophthalmol* 1992; 110:1150-1154.

[32] Khaw PT, Doyle WJ, Sherwood MB et al. Effects of intraoperative5-Fluorouracil or mitomycin C on glaucoma filtration surgery in the rabbit. *Ophthalmology* 1993; 100(3):367-372.

[33] Mazey BJ, Siegel MJ, Siegel LI, Dunn SP. Corneal endothelial toxic effect secondary to fluorouracil needle bleb revision. *Arch Ophthalmol* 1994; 112: 1411.

[34] Howe LJ, Bloom P. Delayed suprachoroidal hemorrhage following trabeculectomy bleb needling. *Br J Ophthalmol* 1999; 83: 757.

[35] Potash SD, Ritch R, Liebmann J. Ocular hypotony and choroidal effusion following bleb needling. *Ophthalmic Surg* 1993; 24: 279-80.

In: Fluorouracil

Editors: A. Longinho and S. Dobreiro

ISBN: 978-1-62081-970-8

© 2012 Nova Science Publishers, Inc.

Chapter VI

IMMUNOSPECIFIC ALBUMIN MICROSPHERES AS DELIVERY SYSTEM FOR CISPLATIN AND 5-FLUOROURACIL FOR THE TREATMENT OF OVARIAN ADENOCARCINOMA

Ernest J. Truter[*] and Aldina S. Santos

Faculty of Applied Sciences, Cape Technikon,
Cape Town, South Africa

ABSTRACT

The dose of chemotherapeutic agents is considered to be a limiting factor in the treatment of cancer. An ideal chemotherapeutic strategy could be to deliver a high concentration of drug that would be released in sustained small amounts from targeted microspheres to effectively kill only tumour cells but yet reduce toxicity to normal tissue. This theory was tested *in vitro* before it was evaluated in a rodent model. We showed that small amounts of drugs were released in a sustained fashion over a two week period. Cells of a rodent ovarian carcinoma cell line were exposed to cisplatin and 5-fluorouracil, either as free drug or encapsulated in albumin microspheres that were either conjugated to monoclonal antibodies or not. Clonogenic and cell survival growth curve assays, as well as micronucleus assays, were used to determine the feasilbility of employing targeted immunomicrospheres as a

---

[*] Correspondence to: Prof. EJ Truter, Faculty of Applied Sciences, Cape Technikon, P.O. Box 652, Cape Town, South Africa.

treatment regimen for ovarian cancer. In cell survival growth curve assays, cell survival was reduced to 1.2% of the control and in clonogenic assays it was reduced to 7.87% when cells were treated with drug-containing immunomicrospheres. 3.2-fold more micronuclei were found in those cells that had been exposed to the drugs in immunomicrospheres than in those subjected to untargeted microspheres. Thus, these results indicate that immunomicrospheres are more effective in delivering cisplatin and 5-fluorouracil directly to the target cells than the unconjugated microspheres. To evaluate this regimen *in vivo*, a DMBA-OC-1R tumour was removed from a Wistar rat and passaged into healthy animals that subsequently developed tumours. 60% of the animals that were treated with 10 mg/kg CDDP and 40 mg/kg 5-FU administered via immunomicrospheres, survived a 90 day time period in comparison to rats treated with 5 mg/kg CDDP and 20 mg/kg 5-FU in its free form. These results suggest that targeted chemotherapy could be an effective option in the treatment of ovarian cancer as high concentrations of chemotherapeutic drugs can be delivered in sustained fashion at the target site with a reduction of systemic cytotoxic side-effects to normal tissue.

INTRODUCTION

Ovarian cancer rates as the second most common gynaecological cancer with one in seventy women being at risk of developing this cancer worldwide. The dismally low survival rate is considered to be as a result of the asymptomatic nature of the disease in its early stages with the result that only 1 in 4 cases are diagnosed before the cancer has spread beyond the ovaries. Platinum-based therapy, either alone or in combination with other drugs is the mainstay of treatment of ovarian cancer, however, greater success has been achieved by administering cisplatin (CDDP) either alone or together with other drugs intraperitoneally than via the intravenous route (Alberts *et al.*, 1996; Ozols and Vermoken, 1997; Morgan *et al.*, 2000). The combination of CDDP and 5-fluorouracil (5-FU) has been widely used in the treatment of different types of cancers including ovarian cancer (Tanaka *et al*, 2001; Harstrick *et al.*, 1997; Neijt, 1996; Braly *et al*, 1995). The synergism of these two drugs has contributed to the increased success rate in the treatment of both human and murine neoplasms (Harstrick *et al.*, 1997; Rooney *et al.*, 1985; Schabel *et al.*, 1979). However when CDDP and 5-FU are used at high concentrations so that treatment can be effective, severe systemic toxicity occurs.

One mechanism by which this problem may be overcome is to make use of a drug delivery system to deliver large concentrations of drug that is released in a sustained fashion. Tamura *et al.,* 2002; Ozkan *et al.,* 2000; Cheng *et al.,* 1993 and Hagiwara *et al.,* 1997 have demonstrated the suitability of human serum albumin microspheres as drug carriers. Conjugating antibodies, specific to tumour cells, to the microspheres can further enhance this mechanism (Poste and Kirsch, 1983). In the process, the amount of drug at the target site will be increased while it is released in a sustained fashion, thus improving the therapeutic index while the effect of the drugs on the non-malignant cells is reduced.

Previous results of MTT assays (Truter *et al.,* 2001) indicated that targeted human serum albumin microspheres (HSAMs) containing cisplatin (CDDP) and 5-fluorouracil (5-FU) were more effective in the *in vitro* cytotoxicity of rodent ovarian cancer cells than non-targeted microspheres.

In this study we confirm that human serum albumin microspheres carrying 5-FU and CDDP and conjugated to monoclonal antibodies to a rat adenocarcinoma cell line, DMBA-OC-1R, produce an enhanced effect of cell kill *in vitro* when compared to unconjugated microspheres and free drug. These results are supported by clonogenic and micronucleus assays. This phenomenon is reiterated in a rodent model where the life span of group of rats treated with immunomicrospheres is prolonged. Animals treated by drug-containing immunomicrospheres had a mean survival time of 60% over a 90 day time period in comparison to 14% over the same time period for those treated with free drugs.

MATERIALS AND METHODS

Materials

Cisplatin and 5-fluorouracil were provided by Farmitalia Carlo Erba. RPMI-1640 medium, 1-ethyl-3-3(3-dimethylaminopropyl) carbodiimide, cytochalasin B and Trypan blue were purchased from Sigma (St Louis, Mo) and Bacto-Difco agar from Difco laboratories. Foetal calf serum (FCS) was obtained from the State Vaccine Institute, R.S.A., penicillin from Intramed (Johannesburg, RSA), acridine orange from Riedel-De Haën and streptomycin sulphate, glutaraldehyde, Total Ionic Strength Adjustment Buffer, Titrisol Platinum Standard solution and dimethyl sulfoxide (DMSO), from Merck (Cape Town, RSA). All chemical reagents were of Analar grade. Human serum albumin was supplied by the Western Province Blood Transfusion Service (Cape Town, R.S.A). Epic oil (Cape Town, R.S.A) donated the cottonseed oil.

Cell Lines and Culture Conditions

Experiments were performed on the rodent ovarian adenocarcinoma cell line, DMBA-OC-1R, which was a gift kindly provided by Dr A. Kataoke (University of Kurume, Japan). The cells were grown in tissue culture dishes (Corning) to a confluent monolayer in RPMI-1640 medium supplemented with 10% (v/v) foetal calf serum, penicillin (50 U/ml) and streptomycin sulphate (20 µg/ml) (hereafter referred to as RP10) at 37°C in a humidified 5% CO_2 /95% air incubator. Aliquots of stock cells in RPMI-1640 with 10% FCS and 10% DMSO were stored frozen in liquid nitrogen. Cells were passaged twice a week by removing the adherent cells with versene (0.77 mM EDTA in buffered saline, pH 7.2). Cell viability was assessed by means of the Trypan blue exclusion method.

HUMAN SERUM ALBUMIN IMMUNOMICROSPHERES

CDDP and 5-FU human albumin serum microspheres were prepared by thermal denaturation at 120°C as described by Truter (1995). The microspheres were lyophilised and stored at 4°C. The initial concentration of 5-FU entrapped in the microspheres was 9373 µg/g microspheres and that of CDDP was 12261 µg/g microspheres. Two IgM monoclonal antibodies, anti-DMBA43 and anti-DMBA93, were raised against antigens on the DMBA-OC-1R cells in our laboratory according to the method of Brown and Ling (1988). These monoclonal antibodies were evaluated to determine their cross-reactivity against various cell lines and were found to cross react strongly with only one (a human ovarian carcinoma cell line) and weakly with two (a human ovarian carcinoma and a human breast carcinoma cell line) out of 16 cell lines (Truter, 1999). They did not react at all with any of the four rat cell lines, both normal and abnormal. The antibodies were coupled to the surface of HSAMs by means of the carbodiimide method of Illum and Jones (1985).

DRUG RELEASE FROM THE IMMUNOMICROSPHERES

Time-course studies were conducted to assess the release of the drugs from these immunomicrospheres. 150 mg 5-FU-loaded microspheres were incubated at 37°C in 3 ml fresh sterile plasma. Leakage of 5-FU and/or its metabolites out of the immunomicrospheres were monitored by sampling the plasma on the first and every second day thereafter for a 14-day period. The leakage of CDDP and/or its metabolites was assessed in a similar manner. For 5-FU assays, 150 µl supernatant of the plasma was added to 450 µl distilled water and filtered through a Millipore filter (pore size = 0.22 µm). Two hundred microlitres of the filtrate was fused with 20 mg sodium hydroxide pellets for 2 h at 500 °C before dissolving in 25 ml distilled water of which 10 ml was mixed with 10 ml of Total Ionic Strength Adjustment Buffer. The fluoride concentration was assessed with a pH meter having an ion selective fluoride electrode. The level of CDDP in the plasma sampled, was assessed by adding 150 µl supernatant of the plasma to 450 µl distilled water and filtering it through a Millipore filter (pore size = 0.22 µm). A calibration curve was constructed using Titrisol Platinum Standard solutions. Twenty microlitres of the filtrate or standard solution was analysed directly in an atomic absorption spectrophotometer (Varian). Absorbance of the platinum standard solutions was plotted against the concentration of the standard solutions. The platinum concentrations of the samples were determined by reading off the value from the graph.

CLONOGENIC ASSAYS, CELL SURVIVAL GROWTH CURVES AND MICRONUCLEI INDUCTION

The *in vitro* cytotoxicity of CDDP and 5-FU was evaluated as either the free drug or in the encapsulated form, by assessing the ability of the treated DMBA-OC-1R cells to form clones in soft agar and by establishing cell survival growth curves *in vitro*.

Treatment of the Cells

In order to assess the cytotoxicity of the synergistic effects of the free drugs, the survival of the tumour cells after 24 h exposure to the free drugs was evaluated as follows: A single cell suspension of DMBA-OC-1R cells was obtained and the cell number (counted with a haemocytometer) was adjusted to 5 x 10^4 cells per 1 ml of RP10 medium. 5 ml of these cells were seeded on 60 mm Petri dishes (i.e. 2.5 x 10^5 cells in total). After the cells were allowed to adhere overnight in a 37°C humidified CO_2 incubator, the culture medium was removed and 5 ml of RP10 medium containing the appropriate amount of drug was added to each dish. Cells were exposed to concentrations (in µg/ml medium) of drugs ranging from 0.01 μg to 1 μg 5-FU and 0.025 μg CDDP. The cells were returned to the humidified incubator for 24h after which time cell cytotoxicity was assessed by means of clonogenic assays and the establishment of cell survival growth curves.

In a separate study we assessed the effects of CDDP and 5-FU that were released from either unconjugated albumin microspheres or immunomicrospheres on the tumour cell line, DMBA-OC-1R. The cytotoxicity of the drugs delivered by this means was assessed only after the cells had been exposed to the drug-loaded microspheres for 5 days since time is required for the drug to be released from the microspheres (Truter *et al.*, 2001). Therefore, after seeding 2.5 x 10^5 cells in 5 ml of RP10 medium per 60 mm Petri dish and allowing the cells to adhere overnight, the cells were washed with RPMI-1640 medium and exposed to the microspheres for 120 h (5 days). The microspheres were resuspended in RP10 medium so that the initial concentration (in μg/ml medium) of encapsulated drugs that were added to the cells was as follows: 10 μg CDDP and either 10 μg or 25μg 5-FU. Cells that had not been exposed to drugs provided the control population in both of the studies (i.e. free and encapsulated drugs).

After exposure to free drugs or encapsulated drugs, the cells were rinsed with RPMI-1640 medium and detached from the surface of the dishes with versene. The detached cells were washed three more times to remove any traces of the drugs. After the final wash, the cell pellet was resuspended in RP10 medium and the number of viable cells was determined by Trypan blue exclusion.

THE CLONOGENIC ASSAY

The cell number was adjusted to 2.5 x 10^3 cells per 1 ml RP10 medium. The cells were seeded in soft agar on top of a feeder layer of 0.5% agar. The feeder layer of agar was prepared as follows: 10 ml of molten 1% agar (Bacto Difco agar) was mixed with 8 ml double-strength RPMI-1640 medium and 2 ml of FCS. 0.5 ml of the agar (final concentration of 0.5%) was added to each well of a 24-well plate (Corning) and allowed to set before the cell/agar layer was added. The cell/agar layer was prepared as follows: 10 ml of molten 1.32% agar (Bacto Difco agar) was mixed with 8 ml double-strength RPMI-1640 medium and 2 ml of FCS (final concentration of agar was 0.66%). This mixture was kept at 42°C until required. 1 ml of cells was mixed with 1 ml of the 0.66% agar mixture. 0.5 ml of the cell/agar mixture was seeded on top of the feeder layer of agar (i.e. 625 cells were seeded). Each dosage sample was set up in triplicate. The plates were incubated for 14 days in a humidified 37°C incubator containing 5% CO_2. The colonies were fixed with 250 µl 3% glutaraldehyde in 0.54% M PBS and scored.

CELL SURVIVAL GROWTH CURVES

Cell survival growth curves were generated in order to study the recovery of the cells after drug treatment. The cell number was adjusted to 1.25 x 10^4 cells per 1 ml of RP10 medium. 2 ml of cells (2.5 x 10^4 cells) was plated onto 35 mm Petri dishes (Corning). 10 Petri dishes per drug dosage was set up. Cell number was assessed at various time points over a period of 168 hours. 2 Petri dishes per drug dosage per time point were counted. The viability of the cells was then determined by Trypan blue exclusion. At each time point the remaining Petri dishes of cells that were still to be counted were fed by removing the old culture medium and adding 2 ml of fresh RP10 medium.

MICRONUCLEI INDUCTION

The presence of micronuclei in a cell is an indicator of chromosomal damage. In order to assess the cytotoxicity of CDDP and 5-FU at the molecular level in DMBA-OC-1R cells, micronuclei were induced. DMBA-OC-1R cells were detached from the surface of two 25 cm^2 culture flasks (Corning) with versene and rinsed with RPMI-1640 medium. After centrifuging the cells at 1500 rpm, a single cell suspension was obtained by resuspending the cell pellet in 5 ml RP10 medium. The cell number was determined by means of a haemocytometer and it was adjusted to 5 x 10^4 cells per ml RP10 medium. 2 ml of the cell suspension (1 x 10^5 cells) was seeded on top of sterile coverslips (22 mm x 22 mm) in 35 mm Petri dishes. The cells were allowed to adhere to the coverslips overnight in a humidified 37°C CO_2 incubator before the drug treatment commenced. The culture medium was removed and 2 ml RP10 medium containing either CDDP, 5-FU or a combination of both drugs (in the free form or encapsulated in albumin microspheres) was added. The cells were exposed for 1 or 24 h to concentrations of 'free' CDDP ranging from 0.005 µg/ml to 0.1 µg/ml and 'free' 5-FU ranging from 0.5 µg/ml to 10 µg/ml. In a separate study, micronuclei induction was assessed in cells that had been exposed for 120 h (5 days) to 5-FU and CDDP that had been encapsulated in albumin microspheres. The initial concentration (in µg/ml medium) of encapsulated CDDP that was added to the cells was 10 µg and that of encapsulated 5-FU was 25 µg. Each dosage sample was set up in triplicate. Cells that were not exposed to the drug provided the control population. After exposure to the drugs, the drug – containing medium was removed and the cells were carefully rinsed with RPMI-1640 medium three times to remove any traces of the drug that had not been taken up by the cell. 2 ml of RP10 medium containing cytochalasin B (Sigma) at a final concentration of 2 µg/ml medium was added to each Petri dish so as to induce mitotic arrest in the cells. The cells were returned to the incubator for 24 h after which the cells were fixed with cold fixative consisting of 3 parts of methanol to one part of acetic acid. After the cells were air-dried, they were stained with 0.001% acridine orange (a nuclear specific stain) in phosphate buffer (pH 6.8) for 1 minute and rinsed five times with distilled water. The coverslips containing the cells were mounted in buffer on glass microscope slides and examined with an Olympus BH2 fluorescent microscope at 495 nm. The nucleation index in each sample was determined and the micronuclei in binucleated cells enumerated.

THE TUMOUR MODEL

Primary, transplantable rat ovarian adenocarcinoma was induced in 10 female Wistar rats, 3-6 weeks old and weighing 40-100 g, by intraperitoneal inoculation of 4×10^6 DMBA-OC-1R cells, suspended in RPMI-1640 medium, using a 27 gauge needle. The tumours were allowed to establish themselves for 14 days in the animals. Abdominal distension due to the accumulation of ascitic fluid was considered to be evidence of reasonably sized tumour-formation. X-rays were also taken to observe for tumour mass formation. The rats were sacrificed by euthanasia and the primary tumours immediately removed aseptically and placed in a sterile Petri dish containing RPMI-1640 medium at 37°C. The tumour was diced into 3 mm^3 cubes which were then transplanted intraperitoneally into 4 groups of female Wistar rats, 4-8 weeks old and weighing 80-120 gm. Tumours were allowed to develop for 10 days in the peritoneal cavities of each animal before treatment commenced. Also, a few 3 mm^3 cubes of tumour tissue were placed in RP10 medium for cell counting. Any fat was trimmed off the tissue. The tissue was minced with a pair of scissors and then placed in a McCartney bottle containing 10 ml of a 0.25% trypsin solution (Difco 1:250) and a magnetic stirrer bar. Digestion took place at 37°C for 20 minutes with slow stirring. Erythrocytes were then lysed with 0.83% ammonium chloride for 5 minutes. The cells were washed twice with RPMI-1640 medium and pelleted by centrifugation at 1500 rpm for 5 minutes. A cell count of the tumour cells was performed using a haemocytometer and RP10 as the diluent.

DRUG THERAPY AND ANIMAL SURVIVAL ENDPOINTS

The drug therapeutic trials in Wistar rats commenced on Day 10 after primary tumour transplantation. Four groups of rats were used. One group (the free drug group) was given an intraperitoneal combined bolus dose of chemotherapeutic agents containing 5 mg/kg CDDP and 20 mg/kg 5-FU. The same dose was repeated 7 days later. The second group (the low dose immunomicrosphere group) was injected intraperitoneally with a combined bolus dose of immunomicrospheres containg 1 mg/kg CDDP and 4 mg/kg 5-FU. The third group (high dose immunomicrosphere group) was injected intraperitoneally with a combined bolus dose of immunomicrospheres containing 10 mg/kg CDDP and 40 mg/kg 5-FU. The reason for doubling the dosage as a bolus dose as compared to the dosage of the free drug group, was that the drug is released slower and in a sustained fashion and can be tolerated well by the animals. This dosage was given to compare the survival rate of this group of rats with those of the low dose immunomicrosphere group. The fourth group, the control group, consisted of rats that were not exposed to drugs. The rats were observed on a daily basis for a period of 90 days and their status recorded. Autopsies were performed on all animals that died. Tissues were removed for macroscopical, as well as microscopical evaluation. After the 90 day period, all surviving rats were killed. Autopsies were performed on these animals and the findings recorded.

STATISTICAL ANALYSIS

All the data are presented as means plus or minus SE. Significance of differences from control values were determined with the Student's t-test and the level of significance was set at $p > 0.05$.

RESULTS

Drug Release from the Human Serum Albumin Immunomicrospheres

The concentrations of drugs that were released *in vitro* were determined in fixed plasma volumes (3 ml) that contained 150 mg drug-loaded monoclonal antibody conjugated or non-conjugated HSAMs (see Materials and Methods). The initial concentrations of the drugs entrapped in the microspheres were: 9373 µg 5-FU/g microspheres and 12261 µg CDDP/g microspheres. These values correspond to 468.85 µg 5-FU/ml plasma and 613.05 µg CDDP/ml plasma. The time-course of the release of the drugs from the immunomicrospheres into plasma at 37° C is illustrated in Fig. 1 (similar values were obtained with the unconjugated microspheres). As shown, there was a progressive time-dependent leakage of the drugs into the plasma. Over the first five days the release rate was relatively slow, showing only traces of 5-FU and CDDP leakage into the plasma. After 5 days, 0.058 % 5-FU was released into the plasma (0.273 µg 5-FU/ml plasma) and 0.015% CDDP (0.091 µg CDDP/ml plasma) respectively. From Day 5 onwards the release rate steadily increased to more substantial levels. Hence, after 9 days the plasma contained 0.635 µg 5-FU/ml plasma and 0.214 µg CDDP/ml plasma respectively. After 14 days, when the experiments were terminated, the accumulated levels of the drugs were: 0.799 µg 5-FU/ml plasma and 0.283 µg CDDP/ml plasma. The rate of release continued progressively and the microspheres had released their total payloads by approximately 30 days (data not shown).

CLONOGENIC ASSAYS

The clonogenicity of DMBA-OC-1R cells in soft agar after 14 days was determined in order to evaluate the long term cytotoxic effects of a fixed dose of CDDP and varying concentrations of 5-FU on the ability of the treated cells to form colonies in soft agar. Cells were exposed to free drugs for 24 h or to drugs encapsulated in HSAMs for 120 h. Preliminary studies confirmed that the cytotoxicity of the individual drugs was dose-dependent (data not shown). This was assessed by means of clonogenic assays and cell growth survival curves. The synergistic effects of 5-FU and CDDP combined is known to be much greater than that of their individual effects (Harstrick *et al.*, 1997; Rooney *et al.*, 1985).

Survival of DMBA-OC-1R cells after 24 h of exposure to 0.025 µg/ml and increasing concentrations of 5-FU declined in a dose-dependent manner (Fig.2a). Only 24.73% of cells that were exposed for 24 hours to CDDP at a low dose of 0.025 µg/ml were capable of forming colonies in soft agar (p<0.05). A significant synergistic effect of CDDP and 5-FU was clearly demonstrated when cells were treated with 0.025 µg CDDP/ml medium and 1 µg 5-FU/ml medium (p<0.05, Fig. 2a).

It is thus clinically possible using a CDDP/5-FU free-drug infusion protocol to produce and maintain cisplatin serum concentrations of 0.025 µg/ml CDDP and 1 µg/ml 5-FU for 24 h with acceptable host toxicity. Therefore the effects of prolonged high-dose CDDP/5-FU exposure on the same cell line, but from a targeted drug delivery system were examined. This was performed in order to examine if the cell sensitivity employing this modality, increased and fell within a clinically achievable range.

Figure 2b demonstrates the effect on the colony-forming ability of DMBA-OC-1R cells exposed for 120 h to immunomicrospheres containing encapsulated drugs. Colony formation was assessed after 14 days. The amount of drugs contained within the targeted HSAMs that was added to the cell cultures initially was 10 µg CDDP/ ml medium combined either with 0, 10 or 25 µg 5-FU/ml of medium. As the leakage of the drugs from the microspheres, as seen in Figure 1 was very slow, the cytotoxicity of the drugs released from the targeting system was only assessed after 5 days in this series of experiments. Therefore as only small amounts of drug are released from the HSAMs within the first five days, the cytotoxicity assessed was that of very low levels of the drugs. After five days, the concentrations of the drugs released by the different HSAMs into the dishes were approximately 0.002 µg CDDP/ml medium, combined with 0.0 µg, 0.006 µg or 0.015 µg 5-FU/ml medium. In an initial trial (data not shown), we determined that the addition of higher concentrations of CDDP caused much tumour cell kill, which made it difficult to demonstrate the synergistic effects of the drugs.

As was observed in Figure 2a, results depicted in Figure 2b also suggest that the addition of 5-FU modulates the effect of CDDP. The addition of 5-FU immunomicrospheres together with CDDP immunomicrospheres not only enhances but emphasises the synergism between the two drugs. When comparing cells treated with 5-FU and CDDP with those only treated with CDDP, a significant difference was observed (p<0.05) (Figure 2b). However, a greater significant difference could be observed when cells treated with 5-FU and CDDP were compared to untreated cells.

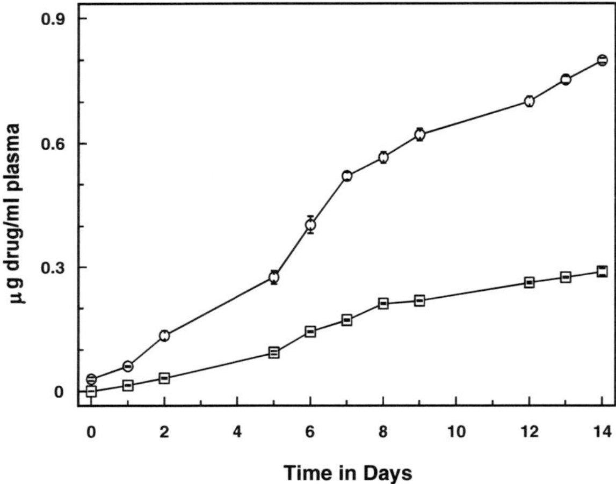

Figure 1. The time-course of the in vitro leakage of CDDP (□) and 5-FU (O) from albumin immunomicrospheres into the plasma at 37°C. Each point represents the mean of at least 5 determinations. Error bars represent the S.E.

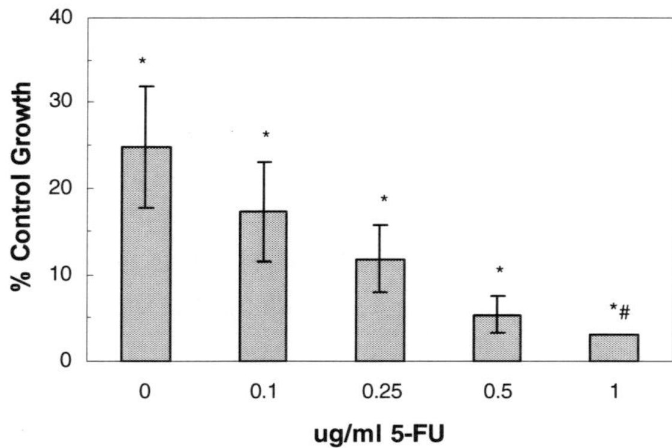

Figure 2a. The clonogenic response of free drug-treated DMBA-OC-1R cells in soft agar. Cells were exposed either to no drugs (control) or to 0.025 µg CDDP/ml medium together either with 0, 0.1 µg, 0.25 µg, 0.5 µg or 1 µg 5-FU/ml of medium for 24 h. They were seeded in agar and assessed for colony formation after 14 days. Data are expressed as a percentage of the number of colonies arising from untreated cells (control cells). Error bars represent SEM (n=3). * = data significantly different from the control population; # = data significantly different from population of cells that were treated only with 0.025 µg CDDP/ml of medium (i.e. no 5-FU was added).

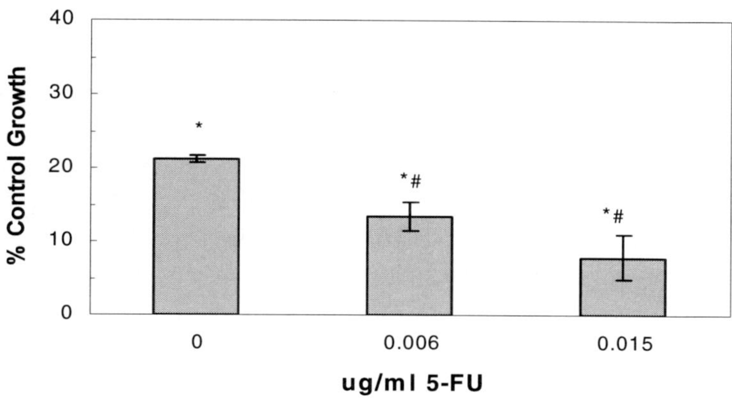

Figure 2b. The clonogenic response of targeted HSAMs-treated DMBA-OC-1R cells in soft agar. Cells were exposed either to no drugs (control) or to approximately 0.002 µg CDDP/ml medium together either with 0 µg, 0.006 µg or 0.015 µg 5-FU/ml of medium for 120 h. They were seeded in agar and assessed for colony formation after 14 days. Data are expressed as a percentage of the number of colonies arising from untreated cells (control cells). Error bars represent SEM (n=3). * = data significantly different from the control population; # = data significantly different from population of cells that were treated only with 0.002 µg CDDP/ml of medium.

CELL SURVIVAL GROWTH CURVES

The cytotoxic effect of a combination of CDDP and 5-FU on the proliferation of cells after treatment was also investigated. As with the clonogenic assays, the cells were exposed to either free drug for 24 h or encapsulated drugs for 120 h. The proliferation of cells that had been exposed to 0, 0.1, 0.25, 0.5 or 1 µg of free 5-FU/ml medium combined with 0 or 0.025 µg of free CDDP/ml medium was monitored over a period of 7 days. A dose-dependent response could be observed when the cells were treated with either 5-FU (Figure 3a) or CDDP (data not shown). The addition of increasing concentrations of 5-FU to 0.025 µg CDDP/ml medium significantly inhibited the survival of cells in a dose-dependent manner (Figure 3a), thereby confirming the synergistic effect of the two drugs observed in the clonogenic assay. After 7 days, the survival of cells that had been treated with 0.025 µg CDDP/ml medium alone was reduced 4.56-fold to 21.95% (Figure 3a). Total cell kill was achieved when cells were exposed to 0.025 µg CDDP/ml medium combined with 1 µg 5-FU/ml medium. This represents another 24.66-fold reduction in cell survival.

Total cell kill was not achieved when cells were exposed to approximately 0.002 µg CDDP/ml medium that had been released from the immunomicrospheres (Figure 3b). Effectively, the cells had been exposed to 400x more CDDP (10 µg/ml medium) encapsulated in HSAMs /ml medium than in the free form. However, as discussed above, the drugs leak out of the microspheres at a very slow rate so that after 5 days the cells have only been exposed to approximately 0.002 µg CDDP/ml medium. Cell death, however, was enhanced by the addition of 5-FU (Figure 3b). Cells were able to recover when exposed to 0.002 µg CDDP/ml medium and 0.006 µg 5-FU/ml medium for 120 h, although it happened at a slower rate than without 5-FU. Cell survival was reduced significantly by 42-fold to 1.2% when the amount of 5-FU to which the cells were exposed was increased to 0.015 µg 5-FU/ml medium (Figure 3b). The efficiency of targeted immunomicrospheres in comparison to HSAMs that have not been linked to monoclonal antibodies against the DMBA-OC-1R cell line, in causing cell death was also investigated (Figure 3c). Untargeted HSAMs had absolutely no growth inhibitory effect on the cells, indicating that immunomicrospheres are more effective in delivering drug directly to the cells than that which are not linked to cell-specific monoclonal antibodies (Figure 3c). There was a significant decrease to 4.03% (Figure 3c) in cell survival when the cells were exposed to the immunomicrospheres for 120 h.

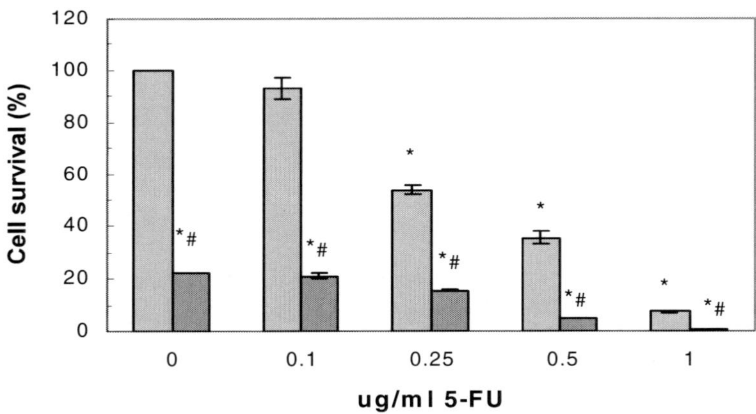

Fig. 3a % Survival of DMBA-OC-1R cells after 168 h of proliferation after 24 h exposure to varying concentrations of 5-FU either on its own ( ) or together with 0.025 µg/ml CDDP ( ). Cell survival was calculated as % of the control cell growth. Error bars represent SEM (n=2). * = data significantly different from the control cell population; # = data ( ) significantly different from the population of cells that was treated with corresponding concentrations of 5-FU only ( ).

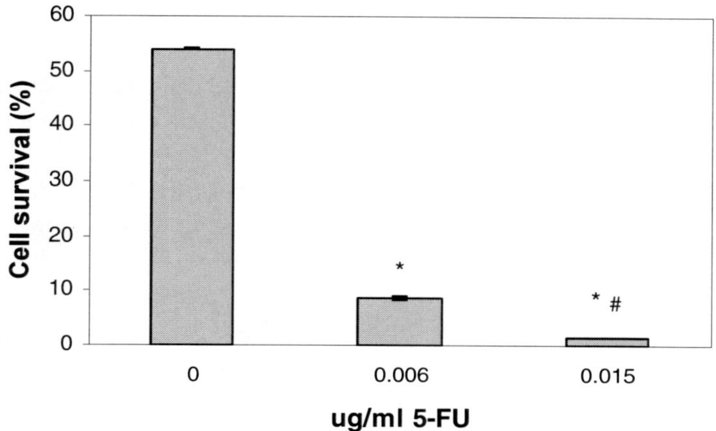

Figure 3b. % survival of DMBA-OC-1R cells after 168 h of proliferation after 120 h exposure to CDDP and 5-FU that had been released from immunomicrospheres. Cells were exposed to approximately 0.002 µg/ml CDDP together with varying concentrations of 5-FU. Cell survival was calculated as a % of the growth of untreated cells. . Error bars represent SEM (n=2). * = data significantly different from the cells that were treated with only 0.002 µg/ml CDDP (i.e. no 5-FU); # = data significantly different from that of the cells treated with 0.002 µg/ml CDDP + 0.006 µg/ml 5-FU.

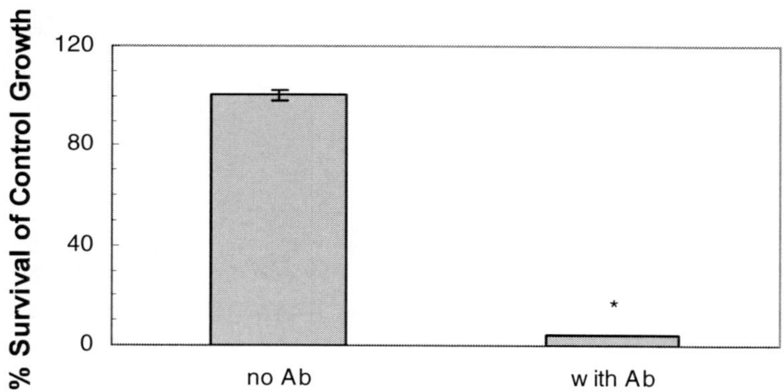

Figure 3c. Effect of CDDP and 5-FU delivered by antibody-targeted and untargeted HSAMs on the inhibition of growth of DMBA-OC-1R cells. Cells were exposed to the HSAMs for 120 h. Cell survival was calculated as a % of the growth of untreated cells (control cells). Error bars represent SEM (n=2). * = data significantly different from the control cell population.

Micronuclei

The mode of action of CDDP is to form intrastrand cross-links in the DNA of cells (Lippard, 1982). Cells, however, are capable of repairing this DNA damage. The inclusion of 5-FU in the treatment regimen is known to inhibit this repair and thereby enhances and ensures cell death. The presence of micronuclei in a cell is an indicator of chromosomal damage. The cytotoxicity of CDDP and 5-FU at the molecular level in DMBA-OC-1R cells was assessed by exposing the cells to either free drug for 24 h or to drugs encapsulated in HSAMs for 120 h. Cytokinesis was blocked with cytochalasin B. The number of micronuclei in binucleated cells was enumerated after the cells had been stained with the nuclear stain, acridine orange. Results are expressed as the number of micronuclei per 500 binucleated cells. The background level of micronuclei in the untreated DMBA-OC-1R cell population was 87.99 ±6.331 (SEM). Cells were exposed to the same concentrations of free 5-FU for either 1 or 24 h (Figure 4a). A significant difference was observed with cells treated with 2.5, 5 and 10 µg 5-FU/ ml medium when the exposure time was increased to 24 h. Significant differences were observed when cells were exposed for 24 h to increasing concentrations of 5-FU. However, these differences were not as pronounced as those observed in the cell survival growth studies, where cells were treated for 24 h with lower concentrations of 5-FU ranging from 0 to 1 µg 5-FU/ml medium (Figure 3a). The effect of 5-FU at the molecular level seems to reach a plateau at 5 µg 5-FU/ml medium. This phenomenon can be ascribed to the fact that 5-FU, unlike CDDP, does not cause DNA strand breakage. A dose-dependent effect was observed in DMBA-OC-1R cells with a 24 h exposure to CDDP with significant increases in micronuclei at concentrations above 0.01 µg CDDP/ml medium. Doses of CDDP greater than 0.1 µg/ml medium resulted in the production of degenerated cells and in increases in the number of multinucleated cells and of micronuclei per cell, which made enumeration difficult (data not shown). The enhancement of cell cytotoxicity by the addition of 5-FU in the treatment regimen, is once again evident in Figure 4b. The frequency of micronuclei increased when 1µg 5-FU/ml medium was added to varying concentrations of CDDP for 24 h. This was especially evident at the lower concentrations of 0.005 and 0.01 µg CDDP/ml medium. The efficiency of targeted immunomicrospheres versus untargeted HSAMs is once again illustrated in Figure 4c. A significant 3.2-fold more micronuclei were found in cells that were treated for 120 h with 0.002 µg CDDP/ml medium and 0.015 µg 5-FU/ml medium that had been released from immunomicrospheres than in those treated with ntargeted HSAMs.

Tumour Model

A rodent tumour model was established in which the activity of the immunomicrospheres could be assessed *in vivo*. Primary transplantable adenocarcinomas were induced in female Wistar rats by injecting 4×10^6 DMBA-OC-1R cells intraperitoneally. Abdominal distension due to the retention of bloody ascites was noted within 10 days of injection. The primary tumours were allowed to establish themselves for 14 days before they were removed, cut into 3 mm cubes and transplanted into the peritoneal cavity of healthy rats. The omentum was the first site in which the tumour appeared following inoculation, after which the tumour disseminated throughout the peritoneal cavity.

The transplanted tumours were allowed to develop into secondary tumours for 10 days before treatment commenced. Tumour mass formation was monitored by X-rays (Figure 5).

The survival of the rats exposed to either the various treatment protocols or rats that did not receive treatment after primary tumour transplantation is depicted in Figure 6. The maximum survival time for the rats that were not treated (Group IIIA) was 19 days. Examination of the peritoneal cavities of the animals who died showed extensive intraperitoneal disease, demonstrating massive hemoascites and peritoneal carcinomatosis with metastases to the liver and spleen. Diffuse studding of tumour deposits on the peritoneal surfaces, viscera and diaphragm was also noted.

Group IA rats (the free drug group) were given an intraperitoneal combined bolus dose as free drugs at a dose of 5 mg/kg CDDP and 20 mg/kg 5-FU, followed by a repeat dose at the same concentrations 7 days later. The free drug was administered twice over a period of a week so as to reduce the effects of the free drug toxicity. Survival studies of this group showed that only 14% of the animals survived the 90-day trial period. All animals that died showed the same peritoneal carcinomatosis as the untreated animals (Group IIIA).

Group IIA rats (low dose immunomicrosphere group) were given an intraperitoneal bolus dose of immunomicrospheres at a dose of 1 mg/kg CDDP and 4 mg/kg 5-FU. This group also indicated that only 14% of the animals survived the 90-day trial period. At post mortem, animals who died showed peritoneal carcinomatosis.

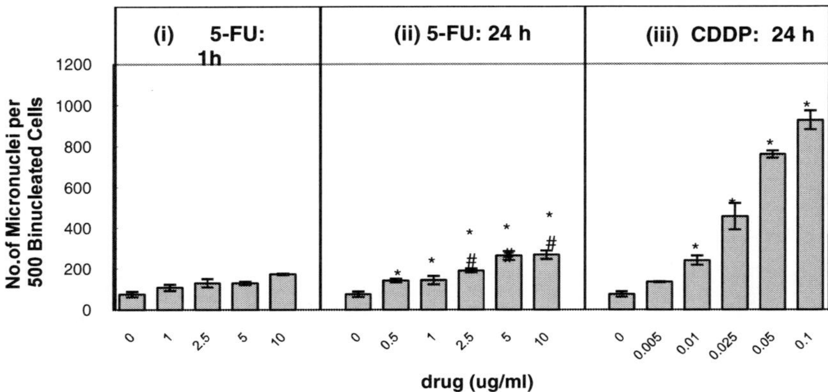

Figure 4a. Micronuclei induction in binucleated cells. DMBA-OC-1R cells were exposed to varying concentrations of either 5-FU for either (i) 1 h or (ii) 24 h or CDDP for 24 h (iii). * = data significantly different from untreated cells; # = data significantly different from that of the cells treated for only 1 h with the same concentrations of 5-FU (p < 0.05). Bars indicate SEM.

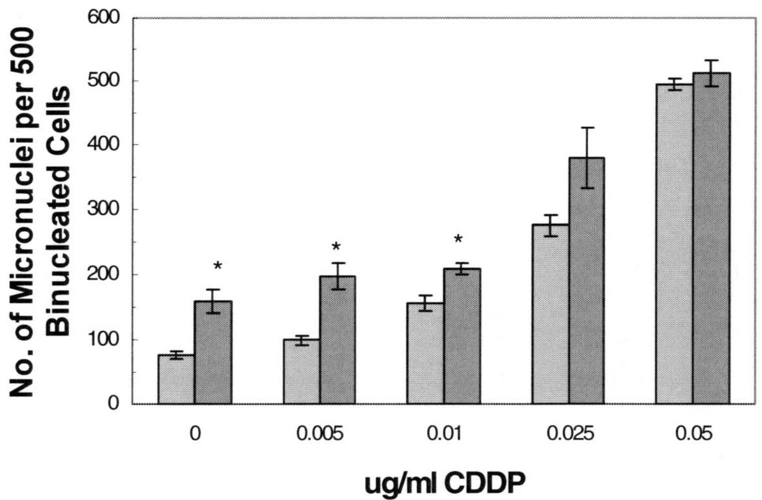

Figure 4b. Effect of the addition of 5-FU in the treatment regimen of CDDP on micronuclei induction in binucleated cells. DMBA-OC-1R cells were exposed for 24 h to varying concentrations of CDDP together with either 0 µg ( ) or 1 µg/ml ( ) 5-FU. * = data significantly different from that of cells treated with only CDDP (p < 0.05). Bars indicate SEM.

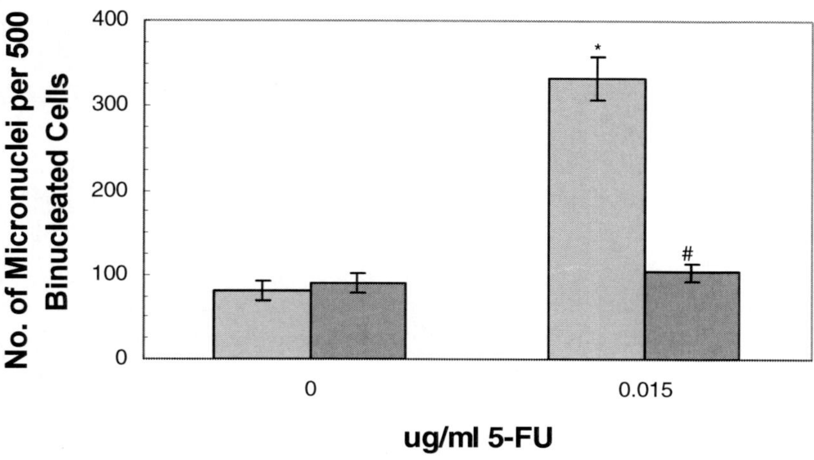

ug/ml 5-FU

Figure 4c. Comparison of the effect of drugs released from targeted ( ) and untargeted ( ) HSAMs on the induction of micronuclei in binucleated cells. DMBA-OC-1R cells were exposed for 120 h to approximately 0.002 µg/ml CDDP together with either 0 µg/ml or 0.015 µg/ml 5-FU. * = data significantly different (p < 0.05) from that of untreated cells; # = data significantly different (p < 0.05) from that of cells treated with targeted HSAMs. Bars indicate SEM.

Group IIB rats (high dose immunomicrosphere group) were given an intraperitoneal bolus dose of immunomicrospheres at a dose of 10 mg/kg CDDP and 40 mg/kg 5-FU. Figure 7 shows drug-containing immunomicrospheres attached to the tumour tissue in the peritoneal cavity. This group of animals showed a markedly improved survival period when compared with the previous treatment protocols with 60% of all animals surviving the 90-day trial period. Again the animals that died showed extensive peritoneal carcinomatosis.

Discussion

Due to the occult nature and high mortality of ovarian cancer, it is considered to be the most deadly of the gynaecological malignancies. Most patients with ovarian cancer require surgery as well as post-operative chemotherapy. The prognosis for women with ovarian cancer that is only diagnosed in the late stages of disease is very poor as at this late stage of disease, the cancer has metastasized to other organs, thus complicating debulking and treatment. The results of several studies have established that platinum-based combination chemotherapy is more effective than single agents or combination of drugs without a platinum analogue in ovarian cancer (Neijt, 1996). Several of the reported regimens include combination therapy with CDDP and 5-FU as they have been shown to exhibit synergistic cytotoxicity against both murine and human neoplasms (Harstrick *et al.*, 1997; Rooney *et al.*, 1985; Schabel *et al.*, 1979). In order to increase the efficacy and therapeutic index of drugs, it would be highly desirable to have delivery systems or techniques that can increase the amount of drug reaching the target site, while reducing the interaction with non-target cells. Particulate drug delivery systems have received much attention as a means of targeting chemotherapeutic drugs to specific sites in, for example, cancer chemotherapy. Albumin microspheres has been described as such a system as it is well-tolerated systemically (Luftensteiner *et al.*, 1999).

We investigated the potential application of tumour targeted albumin immunomicrospheres containing cisplatin and 5-fluorouracil in the treatment of ovarian adenocarcinoma in Wistar rats. Earlier we have shown that the use of monoclonal antibodies to transport CDDP and 5-FU, encapsulated in heat-stabilized albumin microspheres, to tumour cells *in vitro,* creates a feasible possibility for increasing the efficacy of intraperitoneal chemotherapy of ovarian cancer (Truter *et al.*, 2001). Two IgM monoclonal antibodies, designated, anti-DMBA43 and anti-DMBA93 were raised against membrane antigens on DMBA-OC-1R cells (a rodent ovarian cancer cell line) which were used in our studies (Truter *et al.*, 2001). According to Kataoka *et al.* (1987), these cells are morphologically similar to their human counterpart. The specificity of these two anti-DMBA monoclonal antibodies against this cell line was demonstrated in previous studies. We also demonstrated that they can readily be coupled to the surface of CDDP and 5-FU-containing albumin microspheres (Truter, 1999).

These findings indicate that monoclonal antibody-conjugated drug-containing albumin microspheres can be employed as a targetable drug delivery system against rodent ovarian cancer cells. We first tested this hypothesis by investigating whether immunomicrosphere-mediated targeting of CDDP and 5-FU to ovarian cancer cells translates into an enhanced anti-tumour effect compared with non-targeted drug-containing microspheres *in vitro*. The cytotoxicity of the drugs loaded in monoclonal antibody-conjugated albumin microspheres and unconjugated microspheres were assessed *in vitro* in clonogenic, survival growth curve and micronuclei assays.

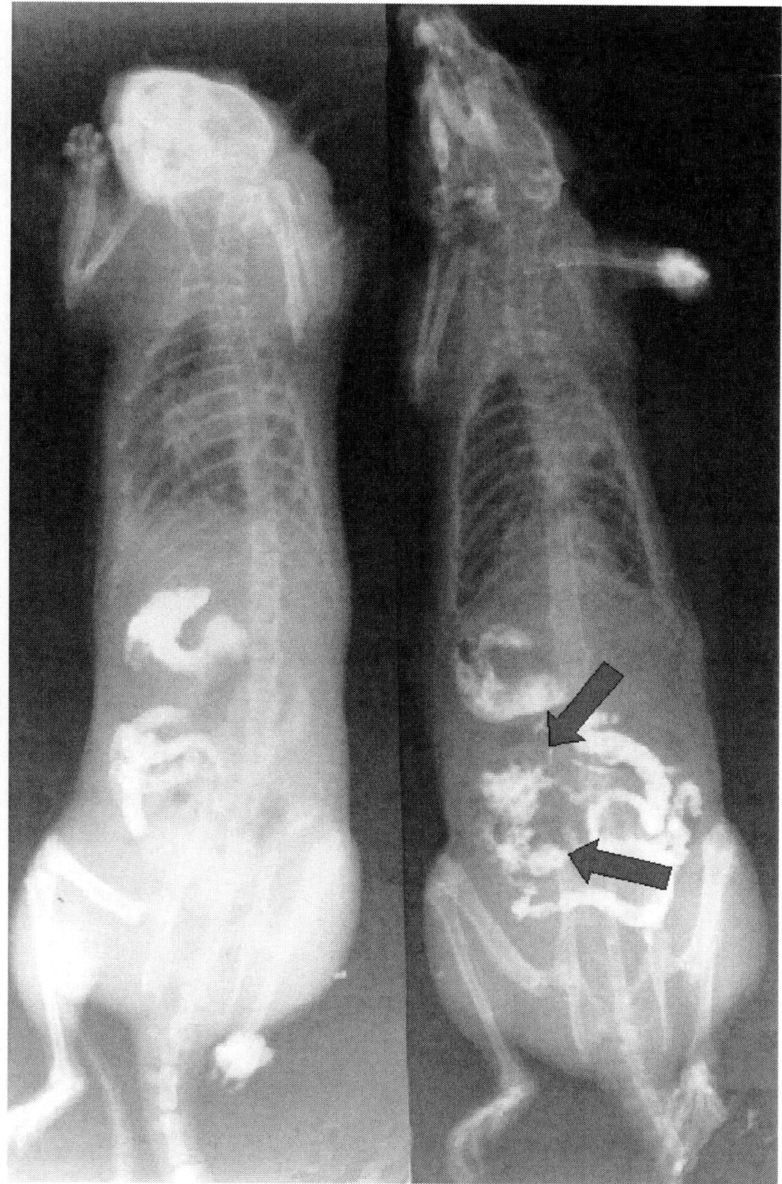

Figure 5. X-rays of control rat (left) without tumour and test rat (right) with secondary tumour mass (indicated by arrows) following intraperitoneal transplantation of 3 mm^3 primary tumour fragment after 10 days (barium contrasted).

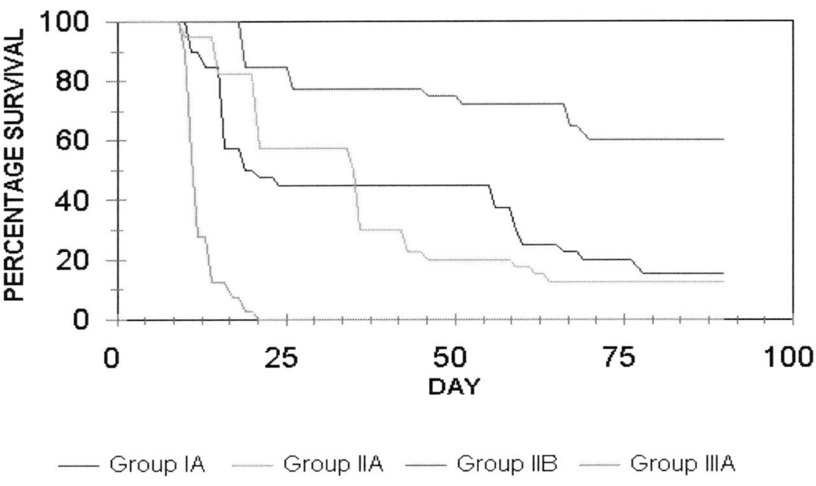

Figure 6. Mean survival curves of animals with transplanted tumours followed by treatment:
Group 1A: free drug group
Group IIA: low dose immunomicrosphere group
Group IIB: high dose immunomicrosphere group
Group IIIA: no treatment group

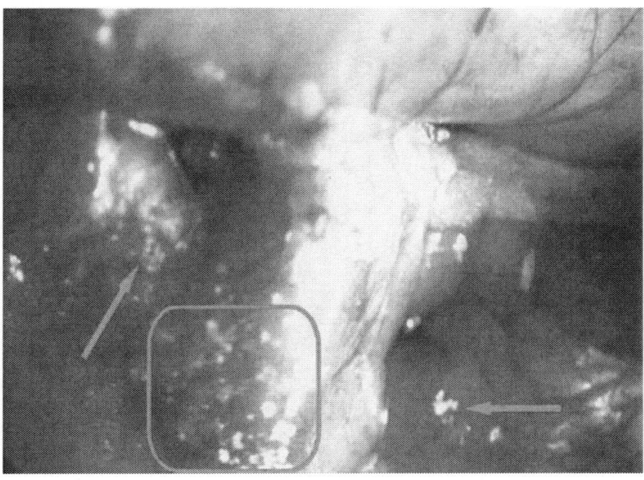

Figure 7. Immunomicrospheres (block and arrows) attached to DMBA-OC-1R tumour tissue in the peritoneal cavity of a female Wistar rat.

Results from the clonogenic assays (Figure 2a) and the survival growth curve assays (Figure 3a), which assessed the ability of cells exposed for 24 h to free drugs, to recover over a period of 14 days (in the clonogenic assays) or 7 days (in the survival growth curve assay), confirmed that the synergistic action of the two drugs was more cytotoxic to the cells than a single agent. The addition of 0.025 µg CDDP/ml culture medium to various concentrations of 5-FU significantly inhibited the cell's growth (Figure 3a). After 168 h, the growth of cells that had been exposed to 0.025 µg CDDP/ml medium and 1 µg 5-FU/ml medium was totally inhibited (Figure 3a).

The aim of targeting drugs to diseased tissue is to deliver a large amount of drug in one bolus dose that can be released in small sustained amounts directly to the tumour cells, thus minimising the toxic effect of the drugs on normal tissue. Thus we compared the cytotoxicity of free drugs to that of the drugs delivered by the immunomicrospheres. Although a total of 10 µg CDDP and 10 µg or 25 µg 5-FU was added per ml of culture medium, the cells had only been exposed to an effective 0.002 µg CDDP and 0.006 µg or 0.015 µg 5-FU/ml culture medium after a period of 5 days. The concentrations of the drugs released from the immunomicrospheres were much lower than that of the free drugs, yet a dose-dependent effect on the cytotoxicity of the cells was still observed (Figure 2b, Figure 3b and Figure 3c). The clonogenicity of the cells was significantly reduced when 5-FU was added in addition to CDDP (Figure 2b). Although cell survival of cells exposed to 0.002 µg CDDP and 0.015 µg 5-FU/ml of culture medium is reduced to 1.2% after 168 h as shown in Figure 3b, we observed that the cells start to recover. This is due to the fact that the microspheres release small amounts of drug and that the microspheres were removed from the cells after 120 h. In the *in vivo* scenario, the microspheres would be in close contact with the tumour cells and would be bombarded constantly by small amounts of drugs that would be released constantly from the microspheres until the microspheres had delivered their full payload. Tumour cells will stand little chance of recovery and should be totally eradicated.

The efficacy of targeted in comparison to untargeted microspheres was also tested *in vitro*. The cytotoxicity of the microsphere system was enhanced when the microspheres were specifically targeted to the tumour cells. Cell survival decreased to 4.03% when the tumour cells were exposed to targeted immunomicrospheres (Figure 3c). Untargeted HSAMs had absolutely no growth inhibitory effect on the cells, proving that a targeted system would be more beneficial in effecting tumour cell kill with minimum toxicity to normal tissue. This result was confirmed with the micronucleus assay (Figure 4c) where 3.2-fold more micronuclei were found in cells that had been exposed to immunomicrospheres than in cells exposed to untargeted microspheres.

The synergistic effect of 5-FU and CDDP whether employed as free drug or released from the immunomicrospheres is reiterated in our results. The results obtained in the clonogenic, survival growth curve and micronucleus assays confirm those results observed with the MTT assay (Truter *et al.*, 2001). Immunomicrospheres containing 5-FU and CDDP are more effective in delivering drug directly to the tumour cells than those which are not linked to cell-specific monoclonal antibodies. Greater cell kill was achieved when CDDP and 5-FU were released in a sustained fashion by immunomicrospheres as compared to cell exposure to free drug. We could thus conclude that a sustained drug delivery system is more effective in delivering its payload to the target site than free drugs.

Based on these results we then tested this regimen *in vivo*. A primary adenocarcinoma was transplanted into healthy, disease-free rats. The presence of tumour in the rats was confirmed by X-rays before treatment commenced. Animal survival curves showed that those treated with the immunomicrospheres had superior survival times compared to those treated with free drugs. Comparative results of rats treated intraperitoneally by a free drug protocol at a dose of 5 mg/kg cisplatin and 20 mg/kg 5-fluorouracil, followed by a repeat dose at the same concentrations a week later showed a survival rate of 14% over a 90 day period. Rats treated with an intraperitoneal bolus dose of immunomicrospheres at a dose of 10 mg/kg CDDP and 40 mg/kg 5-FU showed a survival rate of 60% over the same time interval.

From the above results it was thus possible to extrapolate mortality probability profiles for all 4 groups of animals (Figure 8) used in the survival studies. The results reveal a marked difference in the possible prediction of death of the grouped animals. In the untreated control group (Group IIIA) the probability of death is indicated to be 1 in 3.8 at day 14 after primary tumour transplantation. For rats in the free drug treated group (Group IA), death probability is 1 in 2.1 at Day 72. Death probability for those of the low dose immunomicrosphere group (Group IIA) is 1 in 2.1 while for the high dose immunomicrosphere group (Group IIB) it is 1 in 0.45 at Day 60. This data indicates that the survival probability of animals from Group IIB is substantially superior to the other protocols employed in this study.

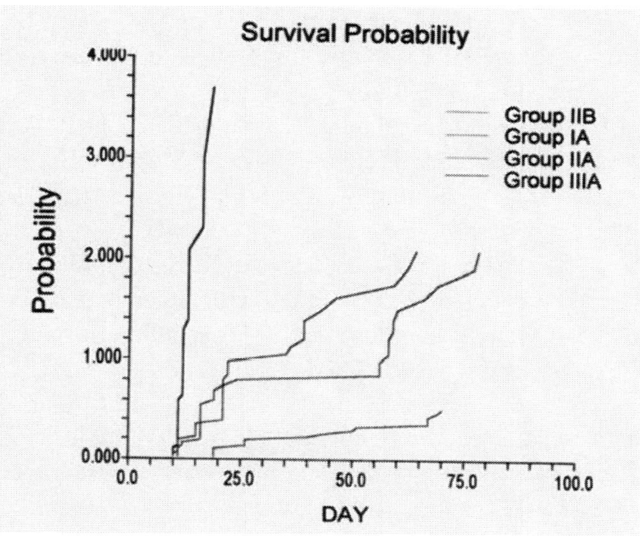

Figure 8. The mortality probability profiles for the groups of Wistar rats:
Group 1A: free drug group.
Group IIA: low dose immunomicrosphere group.
Group IIB: high dose immunomicrosphere group.
roup IIIA: no treatment group.

REFERENCES

[1]   Alberts DS, Liu PY, Hannigan EV, O'Tooles R, Williams SD, Young JA, Franklin EW, Clarke-Pearson DL, Malviya VK, Du Beshter B, Hoskins WJ, Adelson MD, Alvarez RD, O'Sullivan J, Garcia DJ, Sparks DB, Quade J, Rothenberg ML, 1996. Phase III study of intraperitoneal cisplatin-intravenous cyclophosphamide versus intravenous cisplatin-intravenous cyclophosphamide in patients with optimal disease stage III ovarian cancer: A SWOG-GOG-ECOG Intergroup study. *Int J Gynecol Cancer* 6 (Suppl 1): 28-29.

[2]   Braly PS, Berek JS, Blessing JA, Homesley HD, Averette H, 1995. Intraperitoneal administration of cisplatin and 5-fluorouracil in residual ovarian cancer: A phase II Gynecologic Oncology Group trial. *Gynecol Oncol* 56(2): 164-168.

[3]   Brown G, Ling NR, 1988. Murine monoclonal antibodies. In: *A practical approach: Antibodies, Vol 1*. Oxford University Press Ltd., Oxford: 81-104.

[4] Cheng YH, Li L, Fu FH, Liu YY, Liao GT ,Hou SX, Wen YM, 1993. Study on cisplatin albumin microspheres for neck external artery embolization. *Yao Hsueh Hsueh Pao* 28: 604-608.

[5] Hagiwara A, Sakakura C, Tsujimoto H, Imanishi T, Ohgaki M, Yamasaki J, Sawa K, Takahishi T, Fujita T, Yamamoto A, Muranishi S, Ikada Y, 1997. Selective delivery of 5-flourouracil (5-FU) to i.p. tissues using 5-FU microspheres in rats. *Anticancer Drugs* 8: 182-188.

[6] Harstrick A, Vanhoefer U, Heidemann A, Druyen H, Wilke H, Seeber S, 1997. Drug interactions of 5-fluorouracil with either cisplatin or lobaplatin – a new, clinically active platinum analog in established human cancer cell lines. *Anticancer Drugs* 8: 391-395.

[7] Kataoka A, Kojiro M, Yakushiji M, Kato T, 1987. Establishment and morphologic characterization of cell line (DMBA-OC-1) from 7,12-dimethylbenz (a) anthracene-induced rat ovarian carcinoma. *Acta Obst Gynaec Jpn* 39: 842-848.

[8] Illum L, Jones PDE, 1985. Attachment of monoclonal antibodies to microspheres. In: *Methods in Enzymology: Drug and Enzyme Targeting.* Academic Press, New York: 67-84.

[9] Lippard, SJ, 1982 New chemistry of an old molecule. *Science* 4577(218): 1075-1082.

[10] Luftensteiner CP, Schwedenwein I, Eichler HG, Paul B, Viernstein H, 1999. Toxicity of a particulate formulation for the intraperitoneal application of mitoxantrone. *Int J Pharm* 180: 251-260.

[11] Morgan RJ, Braly P, Leong L, Shibata S, Margolin K, Somlo G, McNamara M, Longmate J, Schinke S, Raschko J, Nagasawa S, Kogut N, Najera L, Johnson D, Doroshow JH, 2000.

[12] Phase II trial of combination intraperitoneal cisplatin and 5-fluorouracil in previously treated patients with advanced ovarian cancer: long term follow-up. *Gynecol Oncol* 77(3): 433-438.

[13] Neijt JP, 1996. New therapy for ovarian cancer. *N Engl J Med* 344:50-51.

[14] Ozkan Y, Dikmen N, Isimer A, 2000. Clarithromycin targeting to lung: optimization of the size, morphology and release characteristics of albumin microspheres. *Acta Pol Pharm* 57(5):375-380.

[15] Ozols RF, Vermorken JB (1997). Chemotherapy of advanced ovarian cancer: Current status and future directions. *Sem Oncol* 24(1): Suppl 2: S2-1 - S2-9.

[16] Poste G, Kirsh R, 1983. Site-specific (targeted) drug delivery in cancer therapy. *Biotechnology* 1:869-878.

[17] Rooney M, Kish J, Jacobs J, Kinzie J, Weaver A, Crissman J, Al-Sarraf M, 1985. Improved complete response rates and survival in advanced head and neck cancer after three-course induction therapy with 120 hours 5-FU infusion and cisplatin. *Cancer* 55:1123.

[18] Schabel FM, Trader MW, Laster WR, Corbett TH, Griswold DP, 1979. Cis-dichlorodiammineplatinum (II): Combination chemotherapy and cross-resistance studies with tumours of mice. *Cancer Treat Rep* 63: 1459-1473.

[19] Tamura T, Fujita F, Tanimoto M, Koike M, Suzuki A, Fujita M, Horikiri Y, Sakamoto Y, Suzuki T, Yoshino, H, 2002. Anti-tumour effect of intraperitoneal administration of cisplatin-loaded microspheres to human tumour xenografted nude mice. J Control Release 80(1-3):295-307.

[20] TanakaT, Masuda H, Naito M, Tamai H, 2001. Pretreatment with 5-fluorouracil enhances cytotoxicity and retention of DNA-bound platinum in a cisplatin resistant human ovarian cancer cell line. *Anticancer Res* 21(4A):2463-2469.

[21] Truter EJ, 1995. Heat-stabilized albumin microspheres as a sustained drug delivery system for the anti-metabolite, 5-fluorouracil. *Art Cell, Blood Subs, and Immob Biotech* 23(5): 579-586.

[22] Truter EJ, 1999. Immunospecific albumin microspheres as a drug delivery system for cisplatin and 5-fluorouracil for the treatment of ovarian adenocarcinoma. *PhD thesis,* Department of Anatomy and Cell Biology, University of Cape Town.

[23] Truter EJ, Santos AS, Els WJ, 2001. An assessment of the antitumour activity of targeted immunospecific albumin microspheres loaded with cisplatin and 5-fluorouracil: toxicity against a rodent ovarian carcinoma in vitro. *Cell Biology International* 25: 51-59.

INDEX

Q

R

S

T

U